I wish to dedicate this first volume of the "ASIA" series to Guru Shree Vijayshanti Surishwarji Maharaj, whom I met in India and who gave me peace.

TANTRIK YOGA
HINDU AND TIBETAN

By

J. MARQUÈS-RIVIÈRE
Member of the Asiatic Society

Translated by H. E. Kennedy, B.A.

SAMUEL WEISER
New York

First Published Rider & Co.. 1934
Revised Edition 1970
This American Edition 1970
Fourth Impression 1975

SAMUEL WEISER INC.
734 Broadway
New York, N. Y. 10003

ISBN 0-87728-006-1

Printed in U.S.A. by
NOBLE OFFSET PRINTERS, INC.
NEW YORK, N.Y. 10003

CONTENTS

INTRODUCTION TO THE SECOND EDITION

WHEN J. Marques Riviere wrote TANTRIK YOGA, he was aware of a definite need in the West for the Wisdom of the East. Now, that need has become doubly apparent, but with a vast difference. The West is cognizant of the exigency, and has begun to search for the way out of its stifling ignorance.

Granted a teacher is a necessity, and the tantalizing cliché, "When the pupil is ready, the Guru appears," confronts the Pilgrim. It is to be conceded that there cannot possibly be a guru for each individual. However, that need not deter the determined student, for a knowledgeable book by a dedicated author is an ideal Guru.

Tantrayana has captured the imagination as an illusive subject. It leads us to Tibetan Buddhism where it is interpreted as the perfection of man. As Herbert V. Guenther points out in his THE ROYAL SONG OF SARAHA, ". . . no ceiling is placed on man's capacities."

The nature of Tantrism has been inordinately misunderstood because of the false interpretations placed on it by those in the West seeking emotional outlets. Actually the Tantras were dialogues between Siva, one of the supreme Hindu deities, and Durga, one of the names of Female Energy. Briefly the Tantras were concerned with the creation and dissolution of the worlds. They delved into religion and sought to attain supernatural powers.

One of the most arresting aspects of the Tantras is the terrifying appearances of the deities. Uninformed people have read into these aspects many false conclusions. The actual signification is truly comforting, for the terrifying appearances are assumed by charismatic deities to conquer the powers of evil.

Few Western writers have had the knowledge or the courage to become involved with Tantra. It seems that the symbolism, both erotic and sensual, as well as the amoral teachings have been a protection, making it almost impossible to penetrate into their inner meaning, until the student was ready. Agehananda Bharati, an Austrian by birth, is one of the recent men writing on the Tantra. As an ordained monk of the Dasanami Order of Sannyasi, he received full Tantric initiation. In his book, TANTRIC TRADITION, he elaborates on the subjects that J. Marques Riviere has covered so ably.

Arnaud Desjardins' THE MESSAGE OF THE TI-BETANS, which I was privileged to read in proof, again points to the importance of Tantrayana being rightly understood in the West. It is the logical sequent to Hinayana and Mahayana.

TANTRIK YOGA provides all the requirements for the student. There is an excellent glossary of all the Sanskrit words to allow familiarization with the necessary tools to attack the lessons. The course is laid out in sequence with care and simplicity. The steps are not abruptly presented, but gradually introduced.

When the last page has been turned, it will be found the Guru has lead the seeker through the mysteries of the Yoga and Tantrik doctrines. He will have become aware of the anatomy of the human body according to Yoga. The Chakras and the Kundalini Force are fully explained

—both having long been a matter of conjecture to the average Westerner. The various techniques for the regularization of the breath (*pranayana*) are synthesized, removing all guess work. The *asanas* are described in such a lucid manner, that the correct postures are easily assumed.

Perhaps the most welcome accomplishment is the realization that the correct methods of meditation are no longer complex. The Western student is no longer lost in an incomprehensible atmosphere.

After digesting the contents of this work, the student comes to realize that he has within himself a Living Light —the incomparable Guru who ever waits patiently for the pupil to listen. But the pupil must know *how* to listen. After he has accepted the disciplines (postures and rhythmic breathing) he will KNOW instinctively.

He will understand the Message of the East—THE LIBERATION OF MAN!

Sibyl F.

October 1969

INTRODUCTION

NOBODY can deny that the present is a serious time for the West. The political, social and philosophic values on which the society of yesterday was based have been questioned, one after the other. Some of them have been abolished. Nothing has been spared. The best and the worst meet, strike against one another and recoil. Sometimes they dwell together. Monsters come to birth, monsters scarce capable of living. Ideological social forms transpire, sanguinary struggles take place in this new Middle Age, the Renaissance of which has not yet come in sight.

The domain of the spirit has not been spared, and it is in spirit, perhaps, that men suffer most. One can accustom oneself to ill-made laws, to social insecurity, even to financial instability. One can never accustom oneself to spiritual despair.

What the social planners and reformers have forgotten to do is to give a deep reason for living to those to whom they bring material progress. What do the cinema, television and speed matter, if the soul is dead ? The West has already too long looked like a field of battle, covered with the dying and the dead.

The circumstances of my life have led me to take an interest in the East. The old saying : *"Ex oriente lux"* has impressed me ever more and more. I went to Asia to acquire deep wisdom and peace, from the mouths of men who live there a life which cannot be imagined here.

I shall be told : "You went a long way, whilst at your very door . . ." Ah, there it is—I found nothing at all at my very door, and I am not the only one. My lectures and books on Asia have brought me numerous letters and moving interviews and I have become aware that there is a large public waiting for light and a reason for living amid the stupid life we live.

I do not pretend to a monopoly of wisdom, and the less so since I am only a messenger. The ways that lead to the summit are many. I have come to be aware of one, a marvellous one, and I am showing it to my travelling companions. They will choose it if they wish so to do. . . .

I tell them of my profound faith in the spiritual treasure which the East has retained and the West has lost. This treasure is not occult or secret. Those words, those thoughts I leave to folk who clothe themselves in mystery in order to cloak their ignorance. All that is needed in order to discover the treasure is determination, an ardent desire for the true and the beautiful, and an enduring patience.

Nothing is known of Asia in the West except its political dissensions, which are but the consequences of the lessons we Westerns have given. The deep thought of the East is unknown to us. There are men there whose influence and spiritual authority affect millions. There are mystic forms which satisfy vast numbers of men, but which are almost unknown in the

West. We can no longer remain ignorant of this thought and this culture.

I wish to show you the unknown face of Asia—not by means of recondite treatises, books by learned men, works which only specialists can read ; but by means of texts, commentaries and studies written for all, by means of a living word, a faithful reflection, a message, in brief, from the soul of Asia. The face I will show you will be the face of its spirituality, the living source of that extraordinary mysticism which produces the yogis, sages, mahatmas and lamas, masters of the magic and occult sciences which hitherto have been unexplained in the West.

Liberal eclecticism has guided me in my choice of these texts. I became acquainted with them for the most part during my travels in Asia, when wise men there commented on them for me. No doctrinal or dogmatic considerations have guided me. This is not to be a Jainist or Buddhist, Vedantist or Taoist series. It has not been authorized by anyone. One of the great things I learned in Asia was to reject authoritative spiritual formulae, which limit and often dry up the human heart. I will not, therefore, introduce them here.

My object in presenting these texts to the public is to make people think, reflect. I should be happy if I could awaken attention, give an object to desires, call back a wanderer or satisfy a weary one. But the spiritual life of Asia, while it is poetry and song, is also an extremely subtle psychological technique.

This is the theme of certain texts, which the public does not know, and which will be translated for the first time into a European language for those members of it who are sufficiently interested to read.

I would repeat that I claim no originality for these studies, in which I have but repeated what I have heard. I am but a messenger, who is trying to be not too unfaithful to the Asia whence he comes.

CHAPTER I

A SERIES of works in European languages has at last succeeded in clearing up the serious misconceptions current concerning Asiatic Yoga. It has become known that the word Yoga means something quite different from what it was long thought to mean, and more and more Westerns seek in the mental and physical discipline of Yoga a deep satisfaction in life, and escape from the stifling atmosphere of modern times.

It is necessary, it seems to me, to begin these studies by a succinct and precise exposition of Asiatic Yoga and its teaching. It has often been written that Yoga is an Asiatic "school", "philosophic system", "religious form". So far as I could judge on the spot, the fact was quite different. Yoga is the mystic science of Asia, the accepted basis of all spiritual development, of all religious form.

Everyone who approaches the Asiatic doctrine concerning the various methods of spiritual enfranchisement is struck by the real uniformity which exists under the surface of varying methods of representation. Whatever the kind of physical exercise or meditation, with quick or slow results, whether we have to do with Hindus, with Celanese, Tibetan, or Japanese Buddhists, or Chinese Taoists, the great doctrine of liberation is in its essence identical. Further, it is remarkable that the methods which the Yogis, the "enfranchised", the Taoist masters or the Zens use to prepare the human body are absolutely parallel.

My research concerning the *Tantras* and Tantrik doctrine has proved to me that this knowledge of actions which can transform the human body is part of a science which for want of a better word I will call "esoteric". India was (though China, perhaps, shared the honour) the spiritual master of Asia. To a certain extent it is so still. Hindu missionaries crossed the natural borders of their country and carried the doctrine of the Indian schools all over Asia. Tantrism, the traditional aspect of Yoga doctrine as adapted for our time, has thus been disseminated under varying forms, but always with the same basis.*

That is why the European student is surprised to meet with identical mystic methodologies in Java, Mongolia, China and Japan. The great spiritual current which even in our time runs through the various religious and philosophic groups of the world is the same. It supplies the same needs of the human spirit and, above all, it brings into action the same secret powers of the human body.

The reason of this uniformity of mystic traditions in Asia is comprehensible if we consider that they all aim at the transformation of the human being so that the Divine can effectuate the purpose of creative

* A much larger work, which will appear later, namely, the translation of *The Serpent Power* by A. Avalon, in which I have collaborated with M. Sandor, will set forth the Tantrik doctrines with the greatest precision.

evolution. The presence of the divine in man is coincident with a continuous process of transformation and purification, of elimination of the coarser elements, with a view to the Supreme Identification.

This purification of the human being depends upon physiological knowledge concerning that being, which directs the efforts of the spiritual instructors for themselves and for their disciples. This science of the human body has, however, nothing in common with the anatomical science of the West. Attempts, for instance, to identify the chakras with the plexus are mistaken. He who would reduce everything to terms of the formal, coarse, physical body of man errs here. There is *analogy*, but there is no *localization* or *correspondence*. All that can be said is that the nervous system, acting within the physical body, is symbolically analogous to the complex system of the *nâdîs* and *chakras*, and their action in the subtile body. That is all. But certain Western writers have made the mistake of identifying the solar plexus with the Anâhata chakra, or chakra of the heart. Tantrik doctors in India have pointed out to me that the chakras cannot be identified with parts of the nervous system, as they belong to a quite different plane of "manifested matter".

Thus it is remarkable that in whatever way the tradition is expressed, the process of awakening the centres of subtile energy in the human body is the same. It is even possible to find in Mahommedan tradition very distinct mention of those centres of human energy. Indications concerning them may be found in Sufi and Naqshbandi doctrine, and the Sufis and

Naqshbandis still make use of absolutely "tantrik" methods of realization when working on those subtle centres.* In the Indian Maya tradition of the Sunna (the *Popol Vuh*) there are curious details of the "air tubes" along the spine, which incontestably correspond to the Hindu *nâdîs*. Kundalini is represented by Hurakan, and here the centres of energy are symbolized by animals, corresponding to the deities met with in traditional Hindu descriptions of the centres in a human being.

The sum total of this science of humanity is codified, as one may say, in various texts, of which that by the great Hindu Rishi *Patanjali* seems to be the most esteemed. But he is not unique, and it would be a mistake to think that there is *one* Yoga and *one* method.

The word *yoga* is derived from the Sanscrit root *yog*, which means union or contact. It is, in fact, the science of the union of the human being with the divine dwelling within him. It is the sum of physical, psychical and mental processes which aim at a profound transformation of the human being, the awakening in him of the *new man*, who is transcendental and unattainable by man in his normal state. It is the awakening of new modes of consciousness, of new perceptive faculties, of new powers, the use of which quite transforms that delicate complex which we are.

If the great rules of Yoga are simple, the practical

---

* Al. Birani is said to be the author of a translation of verses in Arabic on Patanjali's "Yoga" written in the seventeenth century.

methods are multiple. It may be said that each individual has *his own* yoga, his exact formula which corresponds to his temperament, to his psychic state, to his atavism, to his past Karma. The great mystic texts of India such as the Bhagavad Gîtâ mention the great divisions of Yoga, known also in the West. They are as follows :

(1) *Hatha Yoga*. *Ha* means the moon and *tha* the sun. This is connected with the two qualities, solar and lunar, of the fluid (prâna) which circulates in the body, and which is directed by the respiratory movement. The regularization of the breath in order to modify the circulation of the prâna or vital fluid is the basis of Yoga. By modifying his prâna the Yogi also acts upon his psychic being, then on his mind, which he modifies in its turn. Thus in the first instance there are *physical exercises*, postures (asanas). This Yoga is essentially Shivaist.

(2) *Râja Yoga*, or Royal Yoga, the mechanism of which is exactly the inverse of the Hatha Yoga. This yoga begins where the Hatha Yoga ends. It works upon the mind with a view to directing the current of the prâna. Mental concentration plays an essential part in it. It is Vishnuist.

(3) *Bhakti Yoga*, or the yoga of devotion, of love for the divine, and of the guru who is its human incarnation. The devotees, the Bhaktis, are, in the presence of their guru, their master, their deity, as it were in the presence of the divine. This yoga is one of the most accessible to Western man, who is already accustomed to the outpourings of the Christian mystic.

(4) *Karma Yoga*, or the yoga of action, subdivided

into an infinite number of yogas. This is the yoga of duty accomplished without affection, without selfishness, without self-interest. It is the great instruction of Arjuna by Krishna in the Gîtâ, when the young prince, on the battlefield of Kurukshitra, hesitates before fighting.

(5) *Jnana Yoga*, or the yoga of knowledge, which is the intellectual realization of the divine, leading to its intuitive realization.

Let us further make mention of the Mantra Yoga, which is the yoga based on the repetition of certain mystic formulas, the mantram, which have a powerful effect upon the subtile bodies of man. It produces the same results as the other kinds of yoga. Then there is *Laya Yoga*, based upon the contemplation of the inward parts (nâda), and produced by closing the ears. I only mention these methods, for in using them without the direction of a master the student is liable to fall into a kind of psychic passivity, absolutely the opposite of the mystic experiences of yoga.

This is an arbitrary classification. As a matter of fact the kinds of yoga interpenetrate one another—nay, are superimposed one upon the other.

The office of the master (guru) is to regulate the exercises and assign the method suitable to the individual disciple. In this the personal factor plays a very great part.

CHAPTER II

THE GREAT BASES OF YOGA DOCTRINE

THE essential problem of life as set by Asia is how to exist and to cease from suffering. Buddhism has made this last the foundation of its thought. The great Rama, the son of Dasharatha, came face to face with this problem, and his guru, the great sage Vasishtha, enlightened his spirit and taught him wisdom by beginning with this: Pain, misery, death and suffering are universal facts for all humanity. They exist everywhere and always. The search for happiness tends towards the extinction of that suffering, which some religious systems have gone so far as to call inextricable from the very web of life itself.

Like Buddhism—which is only a form of yoga—Hindu doctrine affirms that suffering is caused in the first place by desire (vâsanâ, râga, trishnâ). The desire of "the things of the world" is the most dangerous enemy, man's mortal adversary.

But the only reason why we desire the "things of the world" is our ignorance. We do not know the real nature of our inmost being and the relations between things and ourselves. Thus we distort these relations through our ignorance, as Asiatic doctrine enunciates it: "There can be no end to the sufferings of the ignorant man."

Hence we must know ; the only remedy for the sufferings of ignorance is wisdom (jnâna). It is the only possible guide across the ocean of the world. The state of Beatitude, of liberation, *Nirvâna*, in which there is neither death nor birth, is to be attained by knowledge, and by knowledge alone.

By what knowledge ? Not by intellectually attained wisdom, theoretical, bookish science, not by simple quickness of apprehension, but by deep, instinctive knowledge, lived through by the human ego, which is in every man. It is possible to rule the world and not to know peace, if one does not know one's inmost self.

Let us make a brief study (without entering into too great detail) of the way in which Hindu tradition views cosmic construction (the macrocosm) and man (the microcosm). This will enable us to understand the technical bases of Yoga.

The essential principle of Yoga is the existence of the Supreme Principle, Brahma, the unthinkable, the unknowable, the unborn. His activity manifests itself under two aspects :

A positive aspect, masculine, the *Purusha*, the essence of all things, the eternal omnipresent, the creator.

A negative aspect, feminine, the *Prakriti*, the universal plastic principle, the Mother, Isis, the Eternal Virgin, the primordial undifferentiated substance, the root without a root, that which is underneath, that which supports or bears up all manifestation.

In her three forces (*Gunas*) are in action : (1) an ascendant force (sattwa), tending towards more perfect virtue. This is manifested in man when his individuality expresses itself in the form of goodness. (2) A descendant force (*tamas*), darkness, inertia, evil, idleness. (3) An expansive, dynamic force (*rajas*), activity, impulse, desire.

These three *Gunas* exist in different measure in every human being. Their influences are exerted in different ways, and coloured variously by the mind. Thus the sattwic fixes his attention on one sole aspect of things, one sole conclusion, on the possession of a single quality ; the rajasic has pride inherent in his nature, and desires to rule everywhere ; the tamasic seeks for lazy peace, is negative and satisfies himself with the thoughts of ignorance, misery and spiritual incapacity. Yoga aims at the enfranchisement of these three forces.

The action of the Purusha in the Prakriti determines the formation of a vibratory wave in the primordial substance. Differentiation takes place, opposites are defined. Creative waves descend to the lowest degree of manifestation, and thus determine material forms.

Formation of the Human Being

I cannot set forth here the laws and degrees of cosmic manifestation. We now have to deal with the problem of the human being.

Being acted upon inwardly by the *Purusha*, the *Prakriti* encloses or embraces the Purusha, the manifestation of the divine creative will, known in India as ATMA, the indestructible principle of Life, the Spirit

of God, the "specialized", as it were, Divine Presence in
the human being.

But the formation of diverse vibratory waves in the
primordial Substance creates different planes. The
same substance is there ; it "vibrates" differently and
is differentiated into elements which are progressively
"heavier and heavier", until we come to the elements of
our matter.

The human being who above is in direct touch with
the divine has, below, his feet on the "heaviest"
degree of manifestation. He is a complete entity.

These different "matters" (or, rather, vibratory
planes) form multiple envelopes. Each has its peculi-
arity, its differentiation, its qualities. A crude similitude
which is current in India compares them to the scales of
the onion, closely superimposed one on the other. Of
course, there is no superimposition, but more precisely
there are planes of vibration, which interpenetrate one
another. We will study them in the next chapter.

The divine presence (*Purusha*) in the human being
is, and must be, immovable and permanent. The
Purusha is indestructible, for it forms part of the
divine substance and is a direct manifestation of it.

In Hindu tradition the essential ego is called
Paramâtmâ (when regarded from the human point of
view), or Brahma (when it is regarded from a cosmic
point of view). Brahma is neuter, unknowable, without duality, changeless. It cannot be defined or perceived by the human mind. It is the great mystery of
being. Aristotle and the other Greek philosophers
sought to distinguish the attributes and the qualities
of the unknowable, and to describe it. The schools of

Alexandria and Asia Minor preferred silence. In this they were in agreement with the philosophers of India.

Neuter Brahma can only be known through its manifestations, its active and passive, masculine and feminine polarizations, which Hindu tradition calls the Purusha and Prakriti—these two aspects of the undifferentiated, by means of their reciprocal modifications, by reason of the eternal and omnipresent Purusha in the Prakriti, the plastic and substantial principle, determine creation. Under the influence of the Purusha, the essence, the principle of all things, the Prakriti develops, produces entities, multiplies.

The phenomenon is similar on the human plane, and the same hierarchy that orders cosmic "being" orders human beings. The microcosm man is identical with and analogous to the Adam of the Cabbala, the universal man of the macrocosm.

The living soul, the manifestation of Brahma in man, is *jivâtmâ*. The Hindus frequently use the parable of the Sun (the ego, *Atmâ*), which by its ray, Buddhi, makes an image in the water. This image, real for humans, unreal for Brahma, is *jivâtmâ*. This is the manifestation of the *ego* in life, a transitory manifestation and one contingent on Brahma, like all things that reflect the ego and are of the order of a manifestation. It is difficult for a Hindu to conceive the idea of a substance, divine, animating and formative as is its source, but at the same time peccable and fallible. The Hindu thinks as follows: The divine formative energy, the Purusha, is always present in the human being, but human consciousness does not perceive it when it is not liberated by the action (*mâyâ*) of the

Prakriti, which creates the necessary illusion of separateness and individuality.

The Tantriks give to this feminine and passive aspect the name of *Shakti*, and they consider that this aspect is both necessary for creation and forms the obstacle to the "return into God". It is the Consciousness of Being, a Consciousness at once dynamic and static. The Shakti is necessarily dynamic, having the desire to create, to perfect, to accomplish, which is created in her by the Purusha hidden within her. She is necessarily static because she has the illusion of finality, the blindness and stability that are of her very nature. Hindu doctrine, as we have seen, has designated these various cosmic and human forces by the name of *Gunas*, which are three in number : the *Sattva Guna*, which awakens consciousness and perfects creation ; the *Tamas Guna*, which veils consciousness, which is the passive aspect of things ; and finally the *Rajah Guna*, which modifies the excess of both tendencies.

Hindu tradition perceives, finally, three "envelopes" in man : *the causal body* (Kâransharira, or parasharira as the Tantriks call it) ; *the subtile body* (Sûkhsohma-sharîra) ; and the *physical or material body* (Sthûla-sharîra). These envelopes, which enclose the divine presence, Atmâ, proceed, as we now know, from the transformation of the Prakriti by the interior action of the indestructible ferment of the Purusha. But we also know that this aspect of God as Creator (which the Hindus call Ishwara) is not affected by His own creation ; that creation is blind, but the God that dwells in it is awake and awaits unweariedly, admirably for His creature to recognize Him and to realize the deep-seated identity of the human being and all creation with Him.

I will not dwell here upon Tantric metaphysics, I will just point out that the Tantriks, in symbolizing by the Mother the feminine forces which are round about the Purusha, the Shaktis who include and create all beings, make a profound appeal to a living reality in man, which is manifest in all traditions, whether it appear as the great Isis of Egypt, the Asiatic Konan Yn, the Druidic Black Virgin or the Virgin-Mother of Christianity.

This divine presence âtmâ is manifested in the human being by "the ray", of which we were speaking just now, and which is called Buddhi, the principle of the higher intellect, never individualized, and which is higher than the ego-consciousness. This "ray" âtmâ illumines all the individual lower centres. Buddhi is actually the highest principle in the manifestation called humanity. It binds the personality (âtmâ) to its "reflection" (jivatmâ) in the human being. Below, if I may say it, the Buddhi begin the formal states, individualized, the highest of which is Ahamkâra, the sense of individuality. This is created by the action of the outward world upon the world within man. At this stage of manifestation there is sufficient individualization for the elements to be able to act upon it.

This manifestation is afterwards multiplied by the various elements which form the multiple envelopes of the human being.

CHAPTER III

THE SUBTILE ANATOMY OF THE HUMAN BODY ACCORDING TO YOGA—THE NÂDÍS, THE CHAKRAS

WE must now study the various vibratory "envelopes" of the human body.

(1) *The Causal Body*. Form is manifested and actualized by the causal state. This state or condition is formless or universal. Being has no individual existence. It is the sole instrument of real knowledge, for, while undifferentiated, it contains the Purusha and the Prakritî, the whole consciousness (CHIT) of the ego as directed towards its object which is beatitude (ANANDA). This may be schematized as follows :

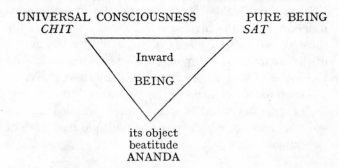

UNIVERSAL CONSCIOUSNESS   PURE BEING
    CHIT   *SAT*

Inward

BEING

its object
beatitude
ANANDA

In this causal state knowledge is apprehended by intellectual intuition, in a certain sense illumination, and not by reflection. Buddhi illumines it directly, since we still have to do with formless manifestation.

(2) *The subtile bodies.* These are called by the collective name of *Linga Sharîra,* and are three in number :

(*a*) *Vijnânamaya kosha,* which directly reflects the Buddhi, the totality of knowledge of the causal body, but which belongs to a coarser order of manifestation, already individualized by Ahamkâra. This envelope is in contact with exterior things through the five tanmâtras, which are the elementary essences or principles of the five senses of man.

(*b*) *Manomaya kosha,* the actual mental body, the kingdom of manas, of the human mind, with its doubts, its processes, its wandering thoughts. The mind is not, for the Hindus, a spiritual faculty. It is one of the faculties of sensation and action, which they call the *indriyas* and which are eleven in number.* The indriyas have a double aspect, being at once physical and psychic. They correspond to the five human senses. This double aspect brings their number up to ten, and if you add the mind, the manas, you get eleven.

The work of the manas is to discriminate between and examine the physical sensations of the five perceptive indriyas, to rule the five indriyas of sensorial action, to imagine, to remember, to understand. To the Hindu his intellect, his manas, *is a sense like the other senses*, which he can modify and render supple. Moreover, as the function of the manas is of the subtile

* The Tantriks "personify" this faculty in deities, and in the Sanscrit letters written in certain figures or mandalas.

order it is exercised by a kind of vibrational accord of the manasic body (or *manomaya kosha*) with the object to be apprehended. Without entering into details which would be useless here, I will just say that, according to Hindu metaphysics, the mind "takes the form of the object which is to be known", so that on the one hand the human being can have only one image in his mind at a time, and on the other hand the intensity of memory and comprehension depends upon the attention given to the object examined, and upon the greater or less capacity of the vibration of the manas to "form itself according to the object studied".

(c) *Prânamaya kosha*. This envelope includes the ten indriyas mentioned above when discussing the manas. They are formed of prâna or vital breath. The prâna also appertains to the subtile manifestation, but by reason of its heavier vibrations it approximates to the physical body, which brings it about that many clairvoyants can perceive the human prâna under the form of coloured vapour. The life-functions which direct the prâna are inseparable from life itself. All the so-called psychic phenomena belong to this domain.

(3) *The physical body*. This is the *Stûla Sharîra*, which is the outer envelope and is composed of the five elements or *bhûtas* : ether or *akasha*, air, earth, fire and water. The flesh is derived from the element of earth, the blood from that of water, the fat, marrow and nerves from the element of fire.

This rapid sketch of the human being must be completed by a description of the three states which man can attain according to whether the vital principle is centred in one or the other of the three envelopes. As a rule the human body is in a waking state (*Vaish-wanara*) ; the human being is then fully conscious of his *ego* (*Ahamkâra*), the sense of individuality. The mind believes that it alone is the supreme Principle and that after its disappearance at death nothing remains. This is due to a great delusion.

Above this state is the *dream state* (*svapna Sthana*), when the *jîva*, the vital principle, retires into the subtile bodies.* Normally this state is attained by human sleep. The exterior world disappears from the consciousness of the human being. The subtile bodies (whose form is similar to or rather "traces" the physical human form) then experience freely the conditions of the subtile planes. These planes of manifestation are as rich and varied as ours. The beings who inhabit them really live; these planes also contain the envelopes of "dead" men which are undergoing what might be translated by the western term "revolution".† This is also called the state of "Taijâsa", or the luminous state. The various psychic phenomena, most supernormal or mystic phenomena of the strange and mysterious life of the beyond, belong to this state, to this intermediate world where man still keeps his limited consciousness, but which is already strictly beyond human space and time (Moksha).

The third state is *the state of deep sleep or sushupta*

---

* We are far here from the "vapours of sleep rising to the brain", by reason of which the organ of touch is immobilized. (St. Thomas Aquinas. *Verit.* q. 12, a.h.)

† At death the subtile bodies dwell in the subtile plane, whilst waiting to resume a physical form. This phenomenon is called *pretyabhâva*, or transmigration (*pretya*, being dead ; and *bhâva*, he who lives anew). There is in this word a sense of death, then of birth, then of death, until Liberation (Moksha) comes.

sthana in which the human being experiences beatitude. This state is only attained by identification with the interior *ego*, the living, immortal *âtma* ; yoga is the way which leads to it. By reaching this state the human being liberates himself from the bonds of the physical and subtile bodies as his consciousness returns to the immutable unchangeable. . . .

.   .

This description of man according to the Hindu tradition will enable us to understand the chapters which are to follow.

The centres of force, the nâdis, belong to the subtile body. The prâna is the vital bond between the physical body and the subtile bodies. It is not the only one. We have seen that the bhûtas (or material elements) also form a bond of this kind, by reason of their double aspect, at once physical and psychical.*

The subtile bodies and the physical bodies are vitalized by the prâna which animates the *Linga Sharira* and corresponds to the astral serpent of Cabbalistic tradition. All living beings, men, animals, deities, only exist in so far as the prâna is in their bodies, either naturally or artificially. For there are rites which give artificial life to an object or to a being recently dead. There is a "breathing-in" of the prâna, a proceeding similar to the charging of an exhausted accumulator with electricity.

But in the human being the prâna circulates in a

---

* The Hindus recognize five states of matter, etheric, gaseous, "free", fluid and solid. The state called "free" is at once burning (tâpa) and luminous (prakâsha).

network of tubes, the nadîs, in just the same way as the cerebro-spinal fluid—*which is not prana, but a much coarser form of the same energy*—circulates in the nervous system, the blood in the veins and arteries, and lymph in the lymphatic system. Hindu physiology takes cognizance thus of another circulatory system, one which is not *closed* or *internal* like the others. Since the prânic system puts the subtile bodies of man (and hence his physical body) in contact with the cosmic prâna, there are centres or openings in the human body through which contact may be established between the human microcosm and the cosmic macrocosm. There is, too, a regulation of the prâna in accordance with the revolutions of the planets and the rotation of the earth. This is that "regulation of the breath" which plays so important a part in Tantrik practice.

As this study is particularly concerned with the centres of subtile energy, we will devote ourselves chiefly to the analysis of the subtile bodies (the *Linga Sharira*). To summarize, the principles which place it in communication with the outside world are as follows :

The five tanmâtras, the essential principles of the five human senses ; the five indriyas of sensorial perception ; the five indriyas ruling sensorial action ; the manas.

This gives a total of sixteen elements, to which must be added the sense of the ego (ahamkâra), elaborated by the manas. This makes seventeen elements in the subtile envelope.*

* I have simplified the Sanscrit terminology as much as possible, and I omit the expository differences between certain schools. Thus the Mâyavâdins replace the five tanmatras by five kinds of prâna. Taking it all in all, it comes to the same thing.

The mechanism of perception is, thus, composed in the following manner : The five objective senses (the five indriyas) are acted upon by the five material elements (the bhûtas). The modification is transmitted to the manas, which perceives, to Ahamkâra, which reacts, and finally to Buddhi, which determines. The mechanism works inversely. Of course there are frequent interferences ; internal or external elements, connected with the subtile planes, falsify, corrupt and divert the process of perception and intuition. This is the "play" of the manifestation, which tends now to "become dull", now to "develop", according to the guna which predominates, as we have already seen.

Besides this material perception, there is continual interchange between the cosmic sphere and the human being. This interchange takes place through the "open centres" of the subtile bodies, and the channels which are made use of for this internal diffusion are the subtile nâdis or "tubes", the luminous arteries which connect on the one hand the various openings corresponding more or less to the natural openings of the physical body. These nâdis, so the texts say, are "woven" into the Linga Sharira like threads into a net. The texts declare that there are a thousand of them. Later on we will study the principal ones.

But there are in this subtile envelope centres where the nâdîs end, which serve at once as regulators and transformers of the prâna. They are centres of consciousness, which work slackly in the normal man, but which can be "awakened" by certain postures and certain concentrations of the manas (mind) upon their activity. This awakening increases their prânic

activity and makes, too, a very great change in the
human being. By the awakening and activity of these
centres of force man acquires powers over the subtile
planes which he had not before. He becomes master
of his subtile bodies as a gymnast becomes master of
his physical body, by the development of certain
muscles. The yogi who consciously awakens these
centres or the mystic who, by an upright and pure life,
by an intense appeal to the divine, awakens them
unconsciously, takes possession in some sort of the
subtile plane, and acquires "gifts" such as clairvoyance
in space and time, levitation, mastery of the physiological instincts (hunger, thirst, sleep, etc.), and it
becomes possible to him to obtain nourishment not by
the absorption of the corporeal elements of foodstuffs,
but by the direct absorption of their prânic or subtile
elements.

This awakening is brought about by the setting in
motion of a new human energy, the *kundalini* force,
which normally lies asleep in the lower part of the
human body, in its lower centre. Kundalini is the
direct image of the divine shakti, of the cosmic power
latent and in repose in man, who can awaken it by
means of certain exercises. It is compared in the
Hindu writings to a serpent unrolling itself, because of
its aspect and its ascent into the great central nâdi of
which we will write later on. The awakening of
kundalini is the sole aim of yoga. Shri Shanka-
râcharya in his Chintâmanistava writes that : "The
bride (the kundalini) entering into the royal way (the
central nâdî) meets and embraces the supreme bride-
groom (Shiva or the divine), and by this embrace they

make floods of nectar flow." This simile gives in brief the mechanism of the awakening of the kundalini force, and indicates that the pure and free activity of this supreme force enables man to realize himself fully as human and as divine, in his body of flesh. There is besides an interior transformation of the essential qualities of the kundalini, gradually as it comes into contact with the centres it awakens.

.   .

THE NÂDÍS

The word nâdî comes from the Sanscrit root *nad*, which means movement. The word may be translated by "tube of subtile force" or "luminous artery". They are all over the subtile body ; their numbers vary according to the tradition of the Hindu schools and the figure is, besides, always symbolic. The Bhûta-shuddi Tantra gives 72,000, the Prapanchasâra Tantra 300,000, the Shiva Samhîtâ 350,000 ; the Prashno-panishad notes 101 principal nâdîs, each with 100 branches, and each of the branches with 72,000. The total is 727,200,000. Their point of issue differs with the differing schools. The Vedantics make them start from the heart, the Yogis from a nerve-centre situated beside the chakra or force-centre near Kundalini.

The prânic currents circulate in the nâdîs, in accordance with very complex rules, governed by the movements of the sun and the moon, the hour of the day, the particular condition of the human being in question, and their own degree of "purity". The "purification

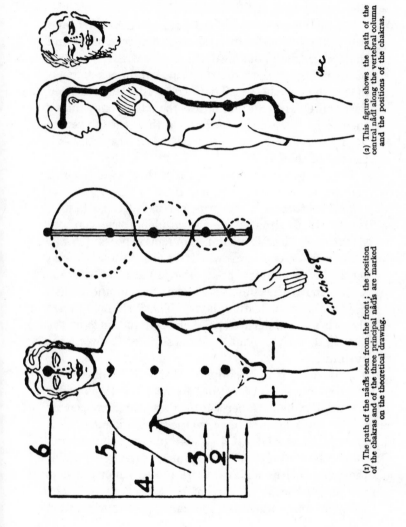

(2) This figure shows the path of the central nâdî along the vertebral column and the positions of the chakras.

(1) The path of the nâdîs seen from the front; the position of the chakras and of the three principal nâdîs are marked on the theoretical drawing.

of the nâdîs" is one of the first important exercises of the yogis. It is called *Shodana*.

Among all these nâdîs there are fourteen chief ones which we will indicate. Of these fourteen there are three which stand out clearly in the Tantrik description of the nâdîs, for these are the principal prânic channels in the human body. They are : Ida, Pingalâ and Sushumna, and Sushumna is the chief one among them. Is is through Sushumna that the power of yoga, the prâna, is forced to pass and to escape through the top of the head.

Here is the description of these three nâdîs, which may be followed on the figures given.

The Sushumna. The principal nâdî of the human being. It is situated in the inside of the cerebro-spinal axis, the Merudanda, and may be said to be next to the spinal marrow. It begins from the lowest centre of the human body, the Mûlâdhâra (situated 5 cm. above the anus and 5 cm. behind the penis). This centre we will study later. The Sushumna passes the other subtile centres, the chakra, and ends at the last of them, the Ajnâ chakra, situated between the eyebrows.

This nâdî is not simple. It is made of subtile matter, composed of various forces ; the three gunas are present in it under the form of three concentric nâdîs : the *nâdî sushumna,* whose predominant guna is tamasic ; the *nâdî vajrâ,* whose guna is rajasic ; and finally the *nâdî chitrinî,* whose guna is sattvic. Then at the centre of the chitrini there is the famous artery, the "royal road", "Brahmanâdî", which is the "tube" through which kundalini passes when it is in motion.

The yogis who have described these nâdîs to me have spoken of them as "tubes", luminous arteries, have spoken of magnificent and changing colour, which varies according to the power and quality of the prâna circulating through them. The texts describe these arteries as "fine as the threads of a spider's web".

The sushumna, then, rises inside the vertebral column, crosses the skull and comes to the chakra situated between the eyebrows, at the lower part of the forehead, below the thousand-petalled chakra (lotus) of the Brahmarandhra. As a rule it does not touch it, but it is quite near it.

The sushumna is uniform, long, straight and erect ; it passes through the six chakras, and, as the Tantrik text has it, "sparkles like a string of jewels". Through it passes the kundalini, the divine force which is the very possibility of liberation.*

The Idâ and the Pingalâ.

Starting from the Mûladhâra like the Sushumna, the two other nâdîs Idâ and Pingalâ also rise towards the chakra in the forehead, but with an inverse, serpentine movement which causes them to pass from left to right and inversely, surrounding each chakra without passing through it like the sushumna.† Idâ is to the

---

* We should mention here a curious Hebrew tradition found in certain commentaries on the *Torah* : God will restore all bodies to life at the end of time by means of the proliferation of an incorruptible and unbreakable bone from the vertebral column. . . . Thus we find an obscured trace of a science of the human body, and a curious analogy between oriental doctrine and rabbinical teaching.

† In this we descry the movement of the two serpents of the Caduceus and the numerous serpentine motives in magical decoration. For instance, it is incontestable that the erected Caduceus at the seat of sex on baphometic idols and on the goats at sabbaths was a degraded indication of a knowledge of the kundalini force.

left : it is the pale and lunar, feminine ; Pingalâ is to the right. It is red, solar and masculine.

In Hindu doctrine these three nâdîs are given the name of the three principal sacred rivers of India. Idâ is the Ganges, Pingalâ is Yamima, and Sushumna is Saraswasti. The Mûlâdhâra, or lower chakra, is the place of meeting of the three rivers (Yuktatrivine). The two nâdîs are bent in the form of an arc, which begins at the fifth chakra and ends in their junction at the Ajnâ chakra, the chakra in the forehead. There they meet for the last time the Sushumna chakra and penetrate it, forming a "triple knot", the Muktatrivinî. From this point the two nâdîs separate again, and the one proceeding from the left penetrates the left nostril, that which comes from the right penetrates the right nostril.

The two nâdîs are the seat of positive and negative activities, constructive and destructive, in accordance with the great cosmic laws. We shall see in a future work the line of march of the prâna to one nâdî or the other, according to the state of the macrocosm. I repeat that it is vain to try to localize the nâdîs, to say that they are situated in one plexus or another, in one sympathetic nerve or another. The most that can be done is to seek a certain correspondence. But the effort of certain doctors, Hindus even, who would see in these traditions primitive lessons in anatomy, are wasting their time. All the Tantriks repeat that these nâdîs are essentially subtile and absolutely invisible to the eyes of the physical body.

But if it is desired to locate approximately on the physical body of man the situation of the chief nâdîs, here is the account given in the Yogarnava and the Sangitaratnakara :

The *nâdî Kuhû* is at the plexus sacrum, to the left of the spine.

The *nâdî gândhâri* goes from the corner of the left eye to the left leg, behind the left sympathetic chain.

The *nâdî hastijihvâ* goes from the corner of the left eye to the great toe of the left foot.

The *nâdî saruswati* follows down the right side of the Sushumna, and ends at the hypoglossic nerves of the cervical plexus.

The *nâdî pûshâ* goes from the corner of the right eye to the abdomen, behind the right sympathetic chain.

The *nâdî pagasvinî* is situated between the two preceding ones.

The *nâdî sankhini* is situated between gândhâri and saraswati.

The *nâdî yashasvini* goes from the right thumb to the left leg, in front of the right sympathetic, following the sciatic nerve.

The *nâdî vârunâ* is between kuhu and yashasvini, in the lower part of the stomach.

The *nâdî vishodarâ* which corresponds to the lumbar plexus, and which also descends towards the lower part of the stomach.

The *nâdî alambushâ* going from the sacral vertebrae to the genital organs.

There are numerous other nâdîs of less importance which the texts do not mention, and which are of no interest.

THE CHAKRAS

Having described the principal nâdîs, we can begin the study of the subtile forces, the *chakras*.

These centres, the general position of which on the Meru (or vertebral column) was given on the figures in the preceding chapter, are called *chakras*, which means "wheels", or *padmas*, which means "lotus". There are six chief ones, which are : *Mûlâdhâra, Svâdhishthâna, Manipûra, Anâhata, Vishuddha* and *Ajnâ.* These chakras are at once the centres of cosmic consciousness, the generators of prâna, and the "openings" on the macrocosm.

I give the figures of the six principal chakras, but oral and written tradition enumerates many more. The full list has no interest for us here, however, for in practice the Tantrik science of the Yoga works only on the six centres indicated above.

Once more we must not hastily localize the chakras anatomically, or seek, as has always been done, a correspondence between them and the various nervous plexus. Analogy, symbolism, yes ! But not identification. I did not find in India any Tantrik really acquainted with the question who maintained this view.

Unless one is a doctor one cannot understand at once that the Tantrik texts, which place the chakras *on the vertebral column* (in the Sushumna nâdî, which transfixes them), cannot place them in the nervous plexus near by. There is coincidence of parallel functions, but the function of the one is exercised on the subtile plane, and that of the other on a much more material plane. The error of anatomically localizing the chakras is of the same kind as that made by modern anatomists and physiologists who think to find "the soul" under their scalpel ; a spiritual or fluidic principle can only be perceived by one who has perceptive senses of the same order as itself. Western science may one day approach the problem of these planes of subtile vibration by means of the use of registering instruments similar to those which it uses for research in connection with electricity, vibrations and air waves.

I will now describe in detail each of the six centres of subtile force, according to the Tantrik books, the principal text among which is the Shat-chakra Niru-pana (description of the six centres of the body).*

Each chakra will be described, the part it plays determined, as well as the psychic forms "controlled" and set in action by its agency.

All the chakras, normally, have the form of a wheel and of a flower. They are upside down except when the kundalini passes over them, when they are right side up.

In principle each chakra is a wheel surrounded by a certain number of petals, and on it is a Sanscrit syllable. This syllable symbolizes, represents, or rather condenses, one or several mystic sounds, the vibration of which more particularly corresponds with the chakra. The sum of these sounds is the *mantra* of the chakra.

The Tantriks add that in the centre of the chakra a Sanscrit letter represents the root (bîja) of the mantra. The forces generated by the centre have, to use a western simile and to avoid the useless accumulation of Sanscrit words, *a fundamental note* and *harmonics*. The bîja, the root-letter at the centre of the chakra, is this fundamental note. The mantra inscribed in the petals corresponds to the harmonics. Moreover, according to the complex theory of colours, essences and sounds, each letter indicates the subtile essence or essences which rule the chakra. That is why each

---

* A precise and literal translation of this text is, beside, in course of preparation by Monsieur E. Sandoz, for the "Asia" Series.

chakra is "coloured" in a particular way, for it contains a subtile energy peculiar to itself.

Finally an animal is indicated in the centre of the chakra, a symbolic animal ; an elephant, a ram, an antelope, etc., as well as a god or goddess. We cannot enter into details which would prolong this summary too much. They will be given later, but I will state here that the symbolic animal described in the text signifies the character of the subtile forces which rule the chakra. The elephant symbolizes strength and stability, and corresponds to the subtile earth-forces ; the ram recalls *ram*, which bears the god Agni, the god of Fire, etc.

The adorned goddesses who are said in the texts to dwell in the interior of the chakras are the *shaktis*, localized divine energies, in some sort contained in the body of every man. The god represents one of the divine forces of the manifestation. Meditation on these forces nourishes them, "awakens" them and sets them working. In their turn these goddesses, these energies latent in the human body, sometimes work unknown to the human being and prepare for or complete the willed work of the transformation of the body.

These indications will enable the reader to understand the descriptions of the chakras which I am about to give.

§ I. MULADHARA CHAKRA (the centre in the lower part of the stomach).

This is situated behind the genital organs and above the anus. Its name is derived from *Mûla* (root) and *adhara* (support) ; it is, as a matter of fact, the root of the nâdî sushumnâ, where the kundalini rests, "swollen like a serpent" ; *it is the real occult centre of the human body.*

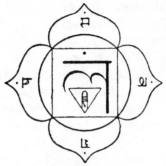

The Mûlâdhâra Chakra.

This chakra has four petals, which are the four forms of beatitude.   Its dominant colour is crimson.

On each petal there is one of the letters : VAM— SAM—SHAM—SAM ; we have seen that this is the mantra of the chakra.   The root (bîja) of this mantra is the letter LAM.   This letter is "seated" on an elephant (Airâvata), symbolizing the terrestrial energies of strength, equilibrium, support and firmness, "shown" also by a yellow square (the earth, *prithivi*), inscribed in the circle.

At the centre of the chakra is a "female" triangle, Yeni, called *traipura*, which is the seat of the lingam, "the male" called Shivalinga (or svayambhu) representing the creative power of Brahma, which is, humanly speaking, symbolized by Kâshi, the city of Benares. Brahma is, too, symbolically seated there on his "vehicle" the swan (Hamsa). Round the linga, luminous as a mass of diamonds, rests, rolled round upon itself three and a half times, the serpentine force kundalini, which concretizes in the subtile sense the life-energy of all animated creatures. Its head covers the orifice of the nâdî sushumnâ.

The goddesses who dwell in the chakras are sometimes called the Queens or Mothers. The Queen of this chakra is the Devi Dakini, who instructs the yogis in the knowledge of the particular energies of this Centre. The Queen who resides in the triangle *traipura* is the Dvi Tripurâ, symbolized by the letter KA, who is evoked by the famous mantra KLIM.

The kundalini lies asleep ; it is the energy which makes the world exist, for it is an aspect of Brahma. The texts say that in sleep the goddess gives vent to a sound similar to the humming of a bee. She is the source of the Word, for from her, by means of successive transformations, the word came forth. She is the Creator and creation in one, the cause of the existence and dissolution of the worlds, the goddess more particularly venerated and loved by the Tantriks.

It is by means of certain meditations that the yogis "awaken" the sleeping Queen. The serpent kundalini then sinks into the nâdî of which it covered the opening, and because of this the divine force awakens in its turn the various centres on its way.

§ II.   SVÂDISHTHÂNA CHAKRA (the genital centre).

Ascending from Mûlâdhâra along the path of the nâdî sushumnâ, the second chakra which one meets is the Svâdhishthâna Chakra.

This chakra has six petals and is of a vermilion colour.

On the six petals are the letters BAM, BHAM, MAM, YAM, RAM, LAM.   This is the mantra of the chakra ; at its centre is the root-letter (bija) VAM.

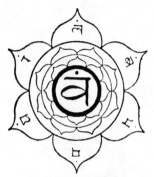

The Svâdhishthâna Chakra.

In the interior of the chakra is the subtile element of water, white in colour, the symbol of which is a crescent (*ardhendu rûpalasitam*) surrounded by eight petals. The bîja *Vam* is also white, "as an autumn moon" says the text, and rests upon a *makara*, a legendary animal which is akin to the crocodile and the sea monster.

The god who "rests" in the bîja of this chakra is Vishnu (or Hari), whose body is blue and who has four arms ; he is seated on his "vehicle" Garuda.

The Mother of the chakra is the shakti Râkini, blue in colour like the lotus of the same hue, of a furious aspect.   Her three eyes are red and one of her nostrils bleeds copiously.

§ III.   MANIPÛRA CHAKRA (the navel centre).

This chakra has ten petals and is grey in colour, similar, as the text says, "to a heavy storm-cloud" (pûrnamegha-prakâsch).

The ten petals have each a letter, in the following order : PAM, PHAM, NAM, TAM, THAM, DAH, DHAM, NAM, PAM, PHAM.*

In the centre of the chakra is the dwelling-place of Fire, the subtile element, represented by an inverted triangle, dazzling like the sun. On the three sides of the triangle are the svastika, and in the middle the root letter (the bîja) of Fire, RAH.

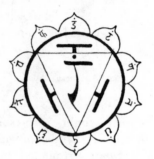

The Manipûra Chakra

This letter rests upon the ram. The god of the chakra is Rudra, covered with white ashes like the Indian ascetics, his hands making the gesture of giving and of removing fear. Rudra is seated on his "vehicle" the bull.

The goddess is the Shakti Lâkini, the universal

---

* As in the other chakras, some of the letters may appear to be similar to each other (DAM and DAM, for instance).

benefactress. The text adds that she loves the flesh of animals, that her breast is covered with the blood and fat which drip from her mouth. This passage is an example of what I said before : that these deities actually represent the various human energies which are localized in the chakras. The fire chakra regulates digestion in the human body. This subtile fire "burns" the food and transforms it, which is why the Mother of the chakra is represented thus. She is blue and is seated on a red lotus, she has four arms and holds the symbols of the ascetics, the Masters of fire.

§ IV. ANÂHATA CHAKRA (the heart centre).

At the height of the heart, on the path of the three principal nâdîs, is the fourth chakra : *Anâhata.*

Its name proceeds from the fact that the Sages can hear from this centre the *sound* (*anâhata shabdu*) which is born in silence, the sound of life. There it is that the vital soul, *Jivâtma*, lives.

This chakra must not be confused with the eight-petalled lotus of the heart, on which one yoga method recommends that the particular deity of the person meditating should be represented, and which is really localized in the heart.

The anâhata chakra has twelve petals, on which are the letters KAM, KHAM, GAM, GHAM, NGAM, CHAM, CHHAM, JAM, JHAM, NYAM, TAM, THAM.

The colour of this chakra is red, similar to that of the flower called Bandhuka.

There is a hexagon at the centre of the chakra ; it is the symbol of Vâyu, or the subtile principle of air ; this hexagon is smoke-grey in colour. In the centre is the root letter (bîja) YAM, the root of the mantra of the twelve petals.

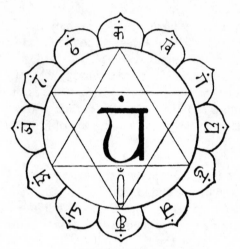

The Anâhata Chakra.

The god who rests in the chakra is Isha, seated on a black antelope, the symbol of swiftness, the vehicle of the subtile elements of the air. The god shines like the sun and he makes a gesture which protects the three worlds.

The goddess is the Shakti Kakini, yellow in colour, benevolent and radiant with joy. Her heart is appeased because she drinks the nectar which the god gives her, the profound symbol of the love which unites the two aspects of the divine manifestation.

In the interior of the hexagon there is a little inverted triangle (trikona) within which is the Shivalinga, shining like a block of gold.   On the top of it there is a little orifice surmounted by a crescent.   The orifice supports the Shakti Lakshmi* under the form of a crescent and a dot.   The god of the linga, Shiva, is symbolized here as animated by ardent sexual desire.

From the centre of this triangle a secondary chakra is projected.   This is the chakra of the heart, which we mentioned before. It has eight petals, and the *Mahanirvana Tantra* calls it *ananda* Kanda.

It is red in colour ; in it the worshipper should picture his familiar divinity, resting under a magnificent tree (Kalpa), surrounded by flowers, fruits and charming birds.

This is not, in the strict sense of the word, a chakra, for it is of an inferior order of subtile activity.

In the *anâhata chakra*, there rests, as we have seen, the vital soul *jivâtmâ*, like a flame, "motionless in space, that has not the least breath of wind"—the symbol of the flame of life which is present in every human being.

§ v.   VISHUDDA CHAKRA (the throat centre).

We find the *Vishudda chakra* at the same height as the throat.   It has sixteen petals on which are inscribed the sixteen following letters : AM, AM, IM, IM, UM, UM, RIM, RIM, LRIM, LRIM, EM, AIM, OM, AUM, AM (anuswara), AH (visarga). The name of the chakra, *Vishudda*, means pure, great, perfect, for by it

---

* Certain meditations on the sexual energies should start from this point, the description of them having been made sufficiently clear.

the vital human soul, the *jiva*, is rendered pure by the vision of *hamsa*, the supreme divine symbol.

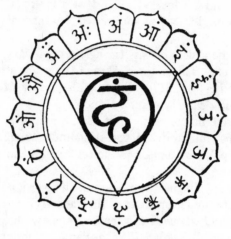

The Vishudda Chakra

Its colour is a smoky purple ; the letters glow red on its petals. There is a white triangle in the centre, enclosing a circle of the same colour with writing in it. This triangle "gleams like the full moon", for this chakra contains the subtile essence of the ether (Akasha).

The root (the bîja) is the letter HAM, set on an elephant. The letter and the animal are white.

The god who dominates the chakra is Shiva (*Sadâshiva*) under his androgynous form (*Arddhanârishvara*), at once male and female. This is symbolized by the golden colour of his left side and the white of his right side.* Without entering into minute details, it is evident that gradually as "one ascends the chakra" the possibilities of acquiring knowledge become more and more extensive. Thus here we come to see the androgynous aspect of the creative god.

The goddess is the Shakti Shâkini, who dwells in this lotus. She is clothed in yellow "luminous in herself", says the text, and she reigns in her lunar region. This corresponds to minor initiation or the little mysteries, major initiation being solar.

The Tantrik text adds, too, that this chakra is the gate of the great liberation for those whose senses are pure and controlled. This Liberation (*Mukti*) is obtained by the awakening of this centre, which enables one to see "the three forms of time", that is, the past, present and future. This text symbolizes the Realization of being beyond time, in the formless manifestation, of which this chakra is in some sort the entrance.

We must note the presence above this chakra, at the base of the palace, of a minor chakra, the *Lalana chakra* (or *Kalâ chakra*, as certain Tantras call it). It is a red lotus with twelve petals.

§ VI. AJNÂ CHAKRA (frontal centre).

Between the two eyebrows, on the forehead, is the last centre of force, *ajnâ chakra*. This name is derived from *ajnâ*, which means rule, for it is in this centre that the yogi receives the orders of his guru.

---

* Here, too, one cannot help realizing the perennial character of Tantrik symbolism in our Western esotericism (Baphomet) ; notably the exact repetition of it in the alchemic Androgyne.

It has the form of a circle adorned with two petals, on which are the letters HA and KSHA. The whole is "like the moon", white and luminous. The two letters sparkle with varied colours. In the centre is the great mantra, the first bîja (or *Pranava*) of the Vedas, the syllable OM.

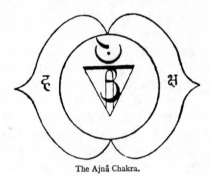

The Ajnâ Chakra.

Shiva is present there in a luminous triangle. He is represented in his phallic form : the Lingua. The triangle symbolizes the feminine yoni. The whole therefore symbolizes the supreme creative act. The text adds that the Lingam sparkles continually in this chakra.

We have seen that three chakras out of six contain the lingam : they are the Mûlâdhâra, the Anâhata and the Ajna. They are looked upon as the three principal chakras in which the powers of the Shaktis, divine energies, are the strongest. The expression "to open the three doors" which is met with in certain rituals, has to do with these three centres.

The queen of this chakra is the Shakti Hâkini, who

has six faces and six arms, which bear certain Tantrik attributes (human skulls, a sacred drum or *damaru*, etc. . . .) She is seated on a white lotus.

The god is Shiva in his creative form, which we have already described. The awakening of this centre is brought about by meditation on these various "presences". We should add that the mind—the *manas*—is situated in this chakra.

It is said that one of the first supersensible manifestations during yoga exercises is a vision of the syllable OM of this chakra, sparkling and radiant like a flame.

Above this centre the Tantrik texts notice two minor chakras : the *Manas Chakra* and the *Soma Chakra.* The *manas chakra* is a six-petalled lotus, which is more particularly the centre of certain psychic phenomena (visions, hallucinations, dreams . . .) ; above is the *soma chakra* with sixteen petals, as well as certain centres where the yogi localizes the spiritual presence of his guru and Shiva.

These "localizations" cross the border of the subtile planes and are not, strictly speaking, centres of force, so I will not dwell upon them lest I uselessly complicate this exposition. These localizations are connected with the causal body and no longer with the subtile planes. I will just enumerate them : above the ajnâ chakra (that is, higher than the subtile forces) is the second Bindu, the creative energy, Shiva ; above this is the Shakti Bodhini ; then Shiva and his Shakti, united, under the form of a crescent moon. Then above the Mother of the Universe, in which all manifestations are dissolved ; then the Shakti Vyâpika, a form of energy which only appears at the beginning of a manifestation ; then Samani and finally Unmani, where supreme realization is effectuated without the aid of the mind. There are seven causal planes corresponding to the seven successive realizations. Arrived at this state says Vishvanâtha, quoting a Tantrik text, there is no longer consciousness or unconsciousness, nor are there any more bodies or gods or time or space.

The final realization is symbolized by the lotus with a thousand petals, the *Brahmarandhra*, the supreme dwelling-place of Shiva, "whiter than the full moon" and with its face downwards. There is a triangle in this lotus, in the middle of which there is "a great void" (*Shunya*), the symbol of the Supreme Light which has no form.

This lotus is above the end of the nâdî sushumna ; the fifty letters of the Sanscrit alphabet are written on each of the thousand petals. Shiva is seated on the *Hamsa*, the symbol of the expiration (Ham), and of the inspiration (*Sah*) of Brahma's breath, which thus manifests itself exteriorly and then manifests itself again (the evolution and involution of the worlds). A description is given in the texts of the various symbols of these states which ascend above the causal planes. It would be useless to give details of them.

.   .   .

We have now come to the end of the description of the six chakras or centres of subtile force in the human body, according to Hindu tradition. The gods, the shaktis, the colours indicated, are not only symbolic ; the Tantriks assert that they can *see* them during their meditation exercises, and that they then become "lived through" experiences, which are related in their texts. These latter are signposts for students who can verify by means of them their own psychic development.

To make this chapter more easily understood, I have drawn up the table on pages 58 and 59 which recapitulates the characteristics of the various chakras.

We should mention here the rather considerable differences between the descriptions found in certain works by a theosophical author, C. W. Leadbeater, and the texts. In a pamphlet published in 1910 and entitled *The Centres of Force and the Serpent of Fire* there are too considerable differences for me to pass them over.*

The situation of the chakras in Leadbeater's work is different. The author places the first chakra at the base of the spine and perceives a cruciform vibration there. The second chakra is situated at the level of the solar plexus ; the third is at the level of the spleen, the fourth, the fifth and the sixth coincide with the texts. There are also great differences as regards the number of petals and the part played by the three

* I would notice for the same reason Sedir's work *The Magic Mirrors*, published in 1907 (p. 16, etc.), which contains a list of the chakras with erroneous names and localizations. The Mûlâdhâra becomes the Maladara ; the Svâdhishthâna becomes Souadosthana ; the Vishudda becomes the Viandha and the Ajna is described as Agneya. The author had not the Tantrik text by him. He assimilates the chakras to the plexus, which is a mistake common to almost all authors who have written about this question. The kundalini becomes the great animating current of the physical body, and as such it belongs to the subtile body, the seat of the mind and consciousness. We have seen that the kundalini in the *normal* human body is dormant, and that its awakening totally transforms the human being who acquires the rank of yogi, of a perfect man.

Name of Chakra	Physical localization	No. of petals	Dominant colour	Geometrical form of the subtile energy	Root letter and its "vehicle"	The God	The Shakti	Letters written on the petals	The subtile force peculiar to each chakra and the sensation activated by its activity
Mûladhâra	Between the anus and the genital organs	4	yellow	square	LAM on the elephant	Brahmâ	Dâkinî	va, sha, sha, sa	*prithivî*, cohesion—energy of smell—rules smell (sensation) and the foot (action) prâna of earth
Svâdhish-thâna	Above and behind the genital organs	6	white	lunar crescent	VAM on the makara	Vishnu	Râkinî	ba, bha, ma, ya, ra, la	*Ap*, contraction—energy taste (sensation) and the hand (for action) prâna of water
Manipûra	At the height of the navel	10	red	triangle	RAM on the ram	Rudra	Lâkinî	da, dha, na, ta, tha, da, dha, na, pa, pha	*tejas*, expansion—heat—energy of colour and form, rules sight (sensation) and the anus (action) prâna of fire

						Isha			
Anâhata	At the height of the heart	12	smoky	hexagon	YAM on the antelope	Isha	Kâkinî	ka,kha, ga,gha, nga, cha, chha, ja, jha, nga, ta, tha	Vâyu, movement in itself—touch—energy of sensation—rules touch (sensation) and the penis (action) prâna of air
Vishuddha	At the height of the throat	16	white	circle	HAM on the elephant	Sadâ-shiva	Shâkinî	the vowels a, â, i, î, u, û, ri, rî, bri, brî, e, ai, o, au, am, ah	Akâsha, spatial energy, energy of hearing—sound—rules hearing (sensation) and the mouth (for action) prâna of ether
Ajnâ	Between the two eyebrows	2	moon-colour	circle	OM (no support)	Shiva	Hâkinî	ha, ksha	Manas, the mind and the energies connected with it.

nâdîs. The author calls sushumna a "force" when it is a nâdî. . . .

Whence come these various descriptions ? Other divergencies are to be found in the English text entitled *The Inner Life*, pp. 443–478, first series. The author has perhaps followed the teachings of another school. We will not judge this question, but will just mention the facts. Our sources are the Tantrik texts, a part of which have been published. Perhaps C. W. Leadbeater has attended different schools. . . . Or perhaps his descriptions come from errors of perception which may be excused owing to the difficulty of the subject and the complexity of this anatomy of the subtile bodies.

CHAPTER IV

THE AWAKENING OF THE KUNDALINI FORCE

I HAVE no intention of describing in detail the various meditations which the texts and oral tradition recommend for the awakening of kundalini. I will not give here more than a few hints which will enable the reader to understand the mechanism. There is a multitude of details about the visualization of gods and shaktis which would weary the reader. These include precise directions for the various forms of meditation, the successive efforts of the mind which are absolutely outside the bounds of this study and will be given elsewhere, in a future work.

The first action required by the Tantrik yoga is the "cleaning" (*shodhana*) of the nâdîs. In order to permit the drowsing subtile forces to pass along the "tubes" and to awaken the sleeping centres, the way must be prepared for the currents to pass, by the psychic purification of the "luminuous arteries" through which the vital fluid, the prana, passes.

This purification is carried out by means of special postures of the body (*asana*), and by breathing exercises (*prânâyama*) ; the mind is habituated to concentrate itself upon a point or an object, real or imaginary, so as to accustom itself to remain calm and to take absolutely "the form" which the will of the yogi wishes to impose upon it. This mental process is concentration or *dhârana*. This concentration brings the mind to be fixed upon one object. This state is technically known as *dhyâna*. When the mind (*manas*) can identify itself with the divine presence in every human being, *atmâ*, it is *samâdhi*.

Let us return to the physical methods used for the awakening of the kundalini force. The yoga particularly adapted for this work is called the Hatha Yoga ; the two syllables *ha* and *tha* mean the sun and the moon and correspond to the movement of the solar and lunar prâna in the nâdîs and to their regulation. Yoga says rightly that the control of the prânic fluid in the human body automatically controls the various activities which the fluid directs and rules.

The purification of the nâdîs (*shodhana*) is carried out by six processes called *Shatkarma*. The description of these latter will be the subject of a book in course of preparation. We will just mention that the Hatha Yoga exercises the intestinal, stomachic and genital muscles, making them work in a peculiar manner, take in, retain and reject air and water. The nostrils and the stomach are cleaned with supple pieces of wood and pieces of linen.

Another purifying process consists of various postures of the body (the asanas), which, the Tantriks assert, automatically clean the nâdîs. In the same way—so I was told in India—as the arm, if raised up, grows white because the blood does not circulate so well in it, a posture correctly adopted regulates certain fluid currents in the nâdîs of the body.

The yogi also uses the *Mudrâs*, certain gestures which accompany the asanas or postures. For instance, in the *yonimudrâ* the yogi, in a squatting position, shuts his anus and pushes the penis back into his body by means of pressure by his feet ; and he shuts his mouth, his ears, his eyes and his nose with his fingers. By means of the mantram *Hum Hamsah* he awakens the kundalini. I will describe the other Mudrâs later on.

The nâdîs having been purified, the Hatha Yoga passes on to the control of the subtile bodies. The control of the breath, *prânâyâma*, is indispensable. Mental control follows the violent breathing exercises, which I will not describe here. These breathing exercises, which strike violently against the diaphragm and in which one nostril or the other is used in accordance with precise rhythm, force, in some sort, the *prâna* to frequent other nâdîs and to awaken the kundalini. There is a whole set of breathing exercises, exterior pressures on the body, muscular contractions, which shut certain nâdîs and waken others. At this stage of realization the yogi makes use of the mantras and the meditations on the centres, the chakra. This is the most interesting part of the matter to be studied, and it is what constitutes in some sort "the secret" of the various schools and the different gurus of Asia. Each master has his particular method. There are those who recommend the way of devotion, the Bhakti yoga, in which the disciple worships the god whom he has chosen, and loses himself in whole-hearted passionate and exclusive devotion. A more peculiarly Tantrik method is to listen to the various sounds of the body, such as the sounds made by the awakening of the chakras and of the kundalini.*

* One curious method consists of stopping the ears and keeping the eyes closed with the fingers, and listening to and contemplating the humming sound which is then audible.

The latter, as we have seen in the description of the chakras, dwells sleeping in the Mûlâdhâra, closing with its mouth the entrance to the sushumnâ. It is imaged with the form of a serpent. This symbolism is universal, and the whole of Asia as well as the ancient Egyptians represents the divine energy under the form of a serpent. The door of liberation is opened by kundalini, the support of the whole human body, the basis of all deep realization, the essence of all yoga. This goddess, this shakti—for the kundalini is considered as a goddess—is the supreme Shakti (*Parashakti*) dwelling in the human body.

The Tantriks make it clear here that sexual energy issues directly from the kundalini. It is, as a matter of fact, logical that human creative force should be derived from the most direct representation of the universal Creative Power. But the whole work of the tantrik yoga consists in bringing it about that sexual force, instead of "descending" under the form of seminal liquid, should retain its subtle form and incorporate itself with the ascending prâna. The *Yoga-Kundali Upanishad** is precise about this : "By the extinction of sexual desire the spirit is freed from its strongest bonds."

---

* The famous text of the *Yoga Vashista* (VI. 80, 36 *et seq.*) gives a description of the centre where the kundalini dwells, which deserves to be quoted here :

"The centre where the goddess rests is circular in form, or like half of the syllable OM. This centre exists in the body of every creature, gods, demons, animals, fishes, birds, insects, etc. In form the goddess resembles a coiled-up serpent, made dormant by the cold. The Kundalini palpitates gently and continually. It is extremely delicate, like 'the pulp of the plantain'. The Kundalini is the greatest, the ultimate power, which orders the life of all animated creatures. It palpitates continually and makes a whistling sound like a furious cobra. Its mouth is open upwards. . . . This Kundalini is also called by divers names according to its functions : *Kâla* for its activity ; *cit* as a manifestation of wisdom ; *jîva* as a synthesis of humanity."

The goddess lies sleeping, and her "expiration and inspiration" maintain the whole body, regularize prâna, are the source of speech. "Her breathing has in it the sounds of all the letters", and that is why, by the universal law of action and reaction, the yogi uses the same letters in the form of a mantra to awaken her.

Normally the prâna ascends and descends along the nâdîs Idâ and Pingalâ and some other nâdîs. The object of all methods is to *empty these two nâdîs of their prâna* and to make them "dead". The prâna is then forced to pass through the central nâdî, the sushumnâ, and thus awaken the kundalini. The normal ascending and descending current of prâna is then troubled to its depths. The various exercises which we have enumerated above have had the result of artificially provoking this "outward march of the prâna", which has the effect of inducing a very great subtle warmth, which warms, too, the yogi's physical body. The serpent kundalini is thus awakened from its state of static equilibrium, and becomes a dynamic force which nothing can stop. A Tantrik said to me : "Can the husband be separated from the wife when they are together ? No ; and neither can the kundalini force be stopped when it has been awakened from its long sleep in the human being."

The kundalini force penetrates into the sushumnâ, the only free way open to it, which leads it to the various chakras and to the goddesses which dwell in them.*

---

* The *Yoga Vashista* thus describes the process: "When the kundalini is filled with prâna (by the joint and abnormal action of the two principal nâdîs) she darts upwards. She then becomes erect and stiff like a stick or an excited serpent. If the various physical orifices are then closed, the body is filled with prâna and its physical and material characteristics are radically changed."

What does the kundalini do with the various centres ? The text says that she "pierces each petal which then rises up erect as she passes". She absorbs into herself the subtile energies (the *tattvas*), corresponding to each chakra, and leaves after her passage her energy alone. In a sense she unifies and exalts the chakra. Her ascent is made from centre to centre, as you have seen, and the centres as it proceeds become more and more subtile.

The lower centres (counting upwards) are associated with the energies of the earth and the water. On the other hand, the succeeding centres contain air and ether. The kundalini repeats inversely the order of the manifestation of the divine energies. The gods and the shaktis are "dissolved" in the great, divine stream, which sets them afire. The mechanism of the dissolution of the subtile energies of matter may be described as the fusion of the elements of these energies in the Sanscrit letter, the root, the bîja which synthesizes them. This bîja dwells in the kundalini current. A thorough transformation of the physical into the subtile is taking place, and of the subtile into the causal, with the help of the cosmic power which creates, sustains and destroys the universe.

This completely interior work is accomplished, as you have seen, by various processes, physical exercises, gestures and breathings, together with concentration and the recitation (or rather singing) of the mantras. The master, or guru, supervises carefully this work of purification and transformation, observing both exterior signs on his disciple and, by direct vision, interior phenomena.

Lists are given in certain texts of the transformations which the awakening of each centre brings about in the human body. There are certain differences in this text. The Shatchakranirûpana enumerates thus the qualities acquired by concentration upon each of the six centres and indirectly by the passing of the kundalini through them :

(1) Meditation on the *Mûlâdhâra* awakens the Shakti and may be considered as the key of liberation and of the spiritual worlds.

(2) Meditation on the *Svâdhishthâna chakra* leads to the mastery of the yogi's "enemies", namely his passions and his selfishness. The passions are ten in number : luxury, anger, greediness, deception, pride and envy, which all proceed from the senses of the individual (*Ahamkâra*). This meditation brings victory over the physical elements.

(3) Meditation on the *Manipûra chakra* gives the power of the destruction and creation of worlds by the mastery of their subtile elements.

(4) Meditation on the *Anâhâta chakra* leads to the mastery of sound—of the word, and thus attains the creative plane of manifestation. The student acquires the faculty, adds the text, of penetrating into the body of other men and animating it in their place, as it was said Shankaracharya did during his life. Other gifts are attained : the power of rendering oneself invisible, of flying in the sky, of walking on water, etc. . . . In a word, the mastery of the planes of creation is complete.

(5) Meditation on the *Vishudda chakra* brings one to the threshold of what the text calls the "Great Libera-

tion". The gods of the subtile planes can no longer attend the yogi, who is beyond the subtile manifestation, for he has attained *"Consciousness of Atmâ"*, that is, he has perceived the supreme identification, the goal of yoga. This is the gist of the long list of qualities and miracles which the texts give when dealing with this state.

(6) Meditation on the *Ajnâ chakra* is the way to the development of the qualities and possibilities of the preceding chakra. Identification which was passive becomes active. The yogi attains the state of Advaita-vâdi where he can see no duality. He becomes the "witness" of the universe.

Other experiences which may be called "mystic" in the western sense of the word come to him then on the causal and formless planes. We will not study them here.

.   .   .

In order to complete this survey we must mention that the Tantriks admit the existence among them of certain Magicians, the *Vâmâchârins*, who know of the existence of the kundalini and the subtile centres, but who deliberately either turn the divine energy from its right path and use it to obtain relative immortality, or for certain human satisfactions, or they stop at certain chakras in order to obtain extraordinary powers and win applause and profit. Certain Tantrik sexual practices proceed from the falsified application of the divine laws.*

---

* I was able to know personally the absolutely depraved and abnormal sexual appetite of these false yogis. The method used is called the Prayoga, through which it is possible to visualize and animate certain female entities who are called *Succubes*.

I must now draw attention to the danger of the premature awakening of the Serpent kundalini in the centre where it reposes. This premature awakening may be caused either by yoga meditations and exercises wrongly done, but advanced sufficiently to awaken kundalini, or by an extraordinary devotion, a fervent bhakti, or perhaps by a physical accident in which the vertebral column is touched. The Serpent kundalini is, we repeat it, of subtile matter, but is so sensitive that a prânic shock on the two great nâdîs stops the normal circulation of the prâna and awakens it.

Yoga is reproached with being a "material and artificial mysticism". The Hindus, as often as I questioned them, have always refused to accept the idea that Yoga was "mysticism" in the Western sense of the word. The word mysticism means etymologically "secret, religious mystery", and mystic theology has used it to describe the ascetic science or art of the supernatural life. But the position of Hindu Yoga must be clearly understood. These exercises, these meditations, these concentrations are not the *aim* of the science of yoga—though certain yogis falsely think that they are—but are the means of attaining to Union which is the real meaning (and even the translation) of the word yoga. Why should there be this mechanical appearance, these complicated processes, this "materialism" in these means ? Because the spiritual science of India—and of Asia as a whole—is quite different from that of the West.

The science of Yoga, the knowledge of the Centres of human force, leading to the mystic realization of the Supreme Identity, proceeds from a quite empirical, quite experimental idea in Hindu asceticism. What I wrote at the beginning of this work about the different conceptions of the human being obtaining in the West and in the East should be recalled. In India, if a supernatural intervention or spiritual beings exterior to man sometimes interfere in human destiny, mystic realization is in the first instance a minute and precise piece of work, an interior transformation. The effort to bring this about requires, of course, the aid of the Divine, but it is in the first instance an awakening of cosmic powers, psychic and mental reintegration into a state which Westerns might call adamic.

From the point of view of oriental asceticism all tends towards the divine, all mystic realization is naturally accompanied by the transformation of the subtile bodies of man and the awakening of the centres of force which "sleep" in him. External or internal circumstances, finally, may delay or hasten this evolution. The method of setting psychic energies in motion is always the same.

CHAPTER V

PHYSICAL METHODS—BREATH CONTROL—MENTAL METHODS

I WILL reserve for a future work the complete and precise description of the physical exercises of Yoga as the texts describe them and as oral tradition prescribes. In this practical exposition of Yoga I wish only to deal with a few Yoga postures which westerns can readily practise.

THE POSTURES OF YOGA (*asanas*)

The preceding chapter should enable us to understand the use of those postures which "clean the nâdîs" and concentrate the mind. The simplest and most practical is the :

Nâsâgra-drishthi. This is the fixing of the attention for a long time on the end of the nose. This sets the optic nerves to work, and should be practised gradually and slowly. Its action on the mind is certain. It calms the mind.

Bhrûmadhya-drishthi. This is the prolonged fixing of the attention on the space between the two eyebrows. The eyes naturally look upwards. These two exercises make the optic nerves work intensively. They are to be practised gradually and calmly. There should be no headaches.

Udhdhiriyâna-Bandha. This is an exercise of the

diaphragm and sides. Its technique may be simply described as follows :

Bandha can be practised either sitting or standing. The student fixes his hands firmly on his knees or on his sides, as the case may be. Having taken up this position, the student breathes out as hard as possible, gradually contracting the interior muscles of the abdomen. The chest is also contracted inwards. Whilst the breath is being held, the neck and shoulder muscles are expanded by the firm pressure of the hands on the knees or on the sides. Then the student tries to inhale slightly, raising his sides and preventing the air from penetrating into his lungs. At the same time the anterior abdominal muscles are completely relaxed.

The three actions which make up the Udhdhiriyâna are, thus, the drawing back of the neck and shoulders, the strong but slight indrawing of the breath, preceded by the greatest possible exhalation of the breath, and the simultaneous relaxation of the contracted anterior abdominal muscles. Automatically the diaphragm rises, and the abdomen is considerably depressed, looking as if there were a hollow. If the trunk is slightly bent forward, the great abdominal concavity becomes yet greater. This position should be maintained during the exercise.

When the student can no longer hold his breath without inconvenience, he relaxes his neck and shoulders, lets go of his sides, and slowly begins to inhale, allowing the abdominal depression gradually to disappear. When it has done so the exercise is finished.

The Padmâsana or Lotus Pose

The Sanscrit word Padma means *lotus*. This pose is called Padmâsana because the hands and feet are so arranged as to imitate the lotus. It may be that the two feet placed upon the opposite thighs represent the leaves, and the two hands placed one over the other the lotus flower.

The student sits down with his legs stretched out as far as possible. He bends his leg at the knee-joint, bends it back upon itself and fixes it in the opposite groin so that the foot is at the root of the thigh, the sole being turned upwards. The other leg is fixed in the same manner. The two heels are so adjusted that they almost unite before the pubic bone, each resting against that part of the stomach with which it is in contact. On the heels, thus united, the student places his left hand, palm upwards. The right hand is then placed on the left in the same manner. The eyes are fixed upon the end of the nose, as we have before described. The technique of the lotus flower is completed by the contraction of the muscles of the anus. It is needless to add that with the exception of the neck, the spine should be held erect.

This asana is illustrated by the pose of the seated and meditating Buddha, which numerous statues have made commonplace in the West.

The Savâsana or Death Pose

Sava, in Sanscrit, means *corpse*. This exercise is called Savâsana because it necessitates a complete relaxation of the muscles, similar to that which takes place at death. In this asana the yogi imitates the position of a dead man.

The technique of Savâsana is easy to understand, but rather difficult to carry out. It is as follows : The pupil lies down on his back and completely relaxes his muscles. It should be remarked that our muscles are always contracted to a certain extent, even when, while awake, we lie down to rest. This slight contraction must be obviated in the death pose. The student must make an effort of will and concentrate a little. He should choose some part of the body and relax the muscles in it. Then he should concentrate his mind on this part and imagine that the whole tissue of the muscle is still more relaxed, quite flabby, as one might say. If he repeats this process constantly he will be able to attain to the complete relaxation of the different muscles.

Generally speaking, one begins with the thorax, then the abdomen, then the lower extremities, then the higher ones, and finally the brain. The eyes should be kept shut. Those, however, who have the strength of will to concentrate while keeping them open may do so, but it is extremely difficult.

While he is endeavouring to relax the different parts of the body the student should at the same time try to act upon several others, so as to be able finally to relax the whole body at once. This complete relaxation is the final aim of the Savâsana.

When the student can relax all the tissues of his body simultaneously he must continue to concentrate on them for some time yet. This completes the first part of the Savâsana. While maintaining the first pose the student must fix his attention exclusively for a second upon the regularization of the respiration, which the Savâsana tends to make rhythmic. This is accomplished as follows :

First phase : The first phase consists of observing the respiration, without trying to control its volume or duration. It should be normal and the observation of it should develop slowly. At the beginning it should be for two or three minutes, then it should be gradually prolonged to ten minutes. During this phase, as during the two following ones, the mind will incline to be easily distracted. Great perseverance over a long period is the only way to attain to concentration.

Second phase : After about a fortnight the student finds that his respiration is irregular, that not only are his inspirations and expirations unequal, but that they lack uniformity. This unequal and irregular respiration is frequently the cause of bad health. Hence it is necessary to correct it. Inspiration and expiration should be of the same duration. The desired regularity should be obtained by prolonging the short or shortening the long. A regular rhythm is all that the student should try to attain. He should exercise for a quarter of an hour daily during this second phase. At the beginning one may have a sense of suffocation, but this soon disappears.

Third phase : At the end of about a month, rhythmical respiration causes a sensation of well-being. The student should then try to increase the volume of the inspiration by breathing in more deeply and in consequence breathing out more. During the whole course of the exercise the mind must be concentrated on the respiratory action.

It is not so easy as one might believe to make one's respiration rhythmic. The most difficult thing is to concentrate the mind. This, however, can be attained with patience. One should not hasten from one phase of the exercise to the other. The second should only be commenced when the first has been mastered, and the third only when the second has been perfectly done.

A great mental effort has to be made in order to attain to rhythm of the respiration, and this effort should only be made with the greatest prudence. Fatigue should always be avoided. The student should never cease to have a sense of well-being and comfort. Even after some practice, nervous persons should not devote more than ten minutes to this exercise, but healthy persons may do it as much as they like, may repeat it twice or even thrice a day.

If well carried out, the Savâsana calms the nerves to such an extent that it is often accompanied by sleepiness, which must be carefully controlled. The student must carefully guard against sleep during his practice of concentration.

Other asanas exist, more and more complicated. I do not think that it would be useful to describe them here. We will refer to them in later studies.

The breath-control exercises mentioned above lead to the *Prânâyâma* or regularization of the breath, which is as important as the postures and which alone can lead to mind control.

REGULARIZATION OF THE BREATH (*prânâyâma*)

There are numerous methods and every yogi has his own. These various techniques may be synthesized thus :

The respiratory movements are classified by the yogi as follows :

(1) *Rechaka*, or exhalation of the breath.
(2) *Kumbhaka*, the pause or stopping of the breath.
(3) *Puraka*, or the inhalation of more air.

The yoga systems lay great emphasis on the pause or retention of the breath. This is a phase which is very important.

The regularization of the breath is brought about by inhaling and exhaling the breath in accordance with a particular rhythm, and through one nostril or the other as determined. Thus one or the other nostril has to be stopped up. In order to do this the yogi uses his right hand. He holds down the index and middle fingers on to the palm, and leaves the thumb, third finger and little finger stretched out. The hand takes naturally the form of the nose, and can stop up one nostril or the other with the thumb or the two fingers.

Here are the progressive exercises essential to prânâyâma :

(1) Stopping up the right nostril with the thumb, inhale slowly with the left nostril and then exhale slowly. Repeat that twelve times.

Stopping the left nostril with the two fingers, inhale slowly through the right nostril and then exhale twelve times each. In this first exercise the breath is not held.

(2) Stopping the right nostril, inhale through the left. Hold the breath. Then, stopping the left nostril, exhale through the right one.

The same thing is then repeated inversely.

But the time of the three movements should be regulated. It should be based upon the figures :

$$1 - 4 - 2$$
$$\text{or } 2 - 8 - 4$$
$$\text{or } 3 - 12 - 6$$
$$\text{or } 4 - 16 - 8 \text{ etc.} \ldots$$

That means that if we take 1, 2, 3, 4, 5, etc., seconds to inhale the air, we must hold our breath for 4, 8, 12, 16, 20, etc., seconds, and exhale for 2, 4, 6, 8, 10, etc., seconds.

In practice the student progresses from 2 to 20 seconds of inhalation and 20×4, equal to 80 seconds, of holding the breath, which is a maximum that should only be attained after some weeks. These breathing exercises must absolutely be progressive.

How should we count ? The Asiatic mind leaves itself free. In practice the measure of time is either the fall of the bead of the Asiatic rosary, the snapping of the finger or heart-beats, or one may count mentally.

(3) The exercise called Ujjagi is more complex. It is done by inhaling through the two nostrils, holding the breath and expelling it through one or the other. The rhythm of this exercise is obtained always as indicated above.

In this last exercise there is usually a snoring sound in the yogi's throat. It is something like the sound of the snores made in sleep. The yogis explain it by saying that it is the vibration of the air in the back of the throat which awakens certain secondary nervous centres.

THE MENTAL METHODS

Besides these physical methods of procedure, the yogi has the mental methods of meditation. Not that he rejects the postures and the breathing, but he requires that the latter should be accompanied by the concentration of the mind and the rendering of it supple.

The unanimous doctrine of Asia about the mind has already been indicated. The *manas* is an instrument of perception, like the five senses, but on a subtile plane. It appertains to a centre of physical activity. It can be unloosed, appeased, purified, calmed. It may be compared—and this comparison is becoming more and more scientifically exact—to a centre continually emitting mental waves.

The mind assembles the activities of the senses ; we perceive things not from without but from *within*. What we see are the modifications of our senses which we perceive and not the things themselves. There is nothing to prove the external reality of our perceptions. A man who always wore green spectacles could not conceive of the universe as other than green. First conclusion : We are enchained by the mental constructions which we are continually creating. If they were extinguished we could apprehend the reality hidden by the play of the mental images which we generate.

We must, too, understand the enormous influence of the mind on the body. Recently medicine has recognized the influence of the mind on physical health. In March 1938, at the last congress held at Hauteville of the doctors from the sanatoria of Jura and the French Alps, several of the specialists adduced singularly disquieting facts. What they told of was as follows : Patients cured of tuberculosis by treatment in a sanatorium, that is to say, having no more trace of lesions as seen by radiography, or of bacilli in their sputum, in spite of long and repeated tests, resumed their occupation and seemed to be in perfect health.

But the mother of one of these patients died of cancer ; another lost her husband ; a third quarrelled with her family, to which she was devoted, because they tried to force upon her a marriage when her affections were otherwise engaged. All three quickly succumbed to a relapse.

Professor Forgue of Montpellier, in an address to the Academy of Medicine, which attracted much attention, spoke of the truly enormous numbers of cancer cases which, since the war, appeared in women who were inconsolable for the loss of a husband or a child.

As regards affections of the heart, there has long been no question. The trouble begins with functional disorder, manifestly nervous in origin. The continued repetition of those disorders in persons who are depressed or haunted by grief finally gives rise to real lesions, taking the form of definite weakness of the myocardis or loss of elasticity in the aorta.

The same could be shown with regard to many diseases of the stomach, troubles and worries affecting in the first instance the appetite, then rendering the stomach and the intestines lazy. This soon reacts on the liver. Hence the case is proved. "A bad state of mind may have a serious influence on the course of disease, even when the disease has an exterior cause, such as the tuberculosis bacillus, and even more when they are conditioned by functional trouble, or when the sympathetic nervous system is the most important factor in them."

These passages from a recent medical work are a confirmation of Asiatic doctrine. The yogi works on the sympathetic nervous system, and his sole method is a mental one.

Patanjali in the *Yogas sûtras* states the basis of Yoga, which is primarily a mental one.

Sûtra 2 : Yogas citta-vritti-nirodhah.

Yoga is the suppression of the transformations of the thinking principle.

Whilst the mind, when free to act, is continually transforming itself and forming itself, better or worse, sooner or later, after the imagined object, Yoga exercises it with a view to remaining motionless and untransformed. For as sûtra 3 of the *Yogas Sûtras* says :

Tadâ drashthuh svarûpe vasthânam.

Then the person seeing (knowing) remains within himself.

Instead of wandering from one mental form to another the yogi retires into himself and can contemplate his EGO. Rab. Tagore has described it perfectly in Sâdhana : "The Supreme vision in our soul is a direct and immediate intuition, which is based neither upon reasoning nor upon proof."

The mind it is that hides reality from us. By its imagination it creates time, space and form. Already Western science (Einstein, Eddington) acknowledges this. But oriental tradition applies this conception of the world to the universe as a whole. It is an ideation (*Kalpanâ-mâtram*) which only exists in the mind and is only an expression of the mind. Everything is an idea, an expression of the mental consciousness.

This creative consciousness has various names. It is often called :

Cid-anu (atom of consciousness) ; or

Manas (absolute activity of consciousness, imagining multiple forms) ; or

Buddhi (fixed on one particular idea and having a definite knowledge of it) ; or

Aham-Kâra (the ego—the sense that "I am") ; or

Citta (a state of quick activity, normal, of reasonless passage from one thing to the other, which is the usual state of the mind).

Manas, say the texts, limits itself like a caterpillar in its cocoon, by the mental forms which issue from it and imprison it.

Further, Asiatic tradition affirms the absolute power of Manas over cosmic construction. The mind, the instrument of creation, is also just as powerful an agent of transformation and destruction. The *Mundaka*

Upanishad declares : "Whatever a pure man desires in his mind and whatever may be his object, he can obtain it" and Asia knows the faith that moves mountains. The Manas is omnipotent. A miracle is a thought clearly expressed.

What the mind imagines intensely can be visualized. The production of ectoplasm by media is an example of this. We build or unbuild our bodies by thought.

Every desire has a tendency to be realized now or later. This is the secret of FAITH.

But our mind is powerful in so far as our thoughts are strong, deep and intense. The yogi's aim is to reinforce Manas by the repetition and constant effort of meditation. The key to Yoga is non-attachment, the suppression of desire, of attachment to the course of life.

Tantrism makes use of numerous methods of calming the "jerks" of the mind and concentrating it. What is essential is to gradually replace the activity of the ordinary reason by that of a force more directly controlled by the Divine. The Tantriks call it the Shakti, the creative reflection of the Purusha in the human being. It should be known that until one has reached the state of deep sleep one can stop the mental transformations but not sensation. The activity of the will should be great enough to act before the ordinary perceptions.

The purification of desire is of the first and greatest importance. The disciple should be free from all desire. But one must beware : impure emotions may "evoke" desire, and Manas may keep them hidden until their next eruption. The will must be strong, the heart pure. Both good and evil desires must be got rid of, to retain only the desire for liberation, which is finally got rid of too.

Yoga distinguishes between the three kinds of desire :

(*a*) Attachment to possessions : this desire must be ignored and not combated.

(*b*) Wish for a thing not in our possession.

(*c*) The like or dislike of certain things ; this should disappear. Indifference must be attained, so that we neither reject nor hold by what belongs to us.

Yoga requires, after the purification from desire (*sumtosa*), calm and the mastery of the senses (*shama*) ; the one as a rule accompanies the other. Then it requires the student to seek the company of the Wise (*sâdhu-sanga*), whose example, whose teachings, whose holy presence help him greatly. Fourthly and finally, Yoga requires *vicâra*, the education of the mind.

MEDITATIONS (*dhyâna*)

The technique of meditation would require a volume to itself. The essential thing is to calm the mind so as to be able to centre the consciousness beyond its activity.

There are "formal" meditations (*saguna*) and "formless" (*nirguna*). The former are based on a mental image, the latter tend to create a mental void.

Patanjali's text is clear (Section III, 1, 2, 3, etc.) :

"Contemplation (*dhârana*) is the fixing of the mind on something."

The unity of the mind with the object of contemplation is absorption (*dhyâna*) or meditation.

When the consciousness has become one with the object contemplated a state of trance (*samâdhi*) is reached.

Yoga, therefore, strives to accustom the mind to concentrate earnestly and completely upon an object, at first material, then imagined. This object or form is chosen with a view to its power to act on the human being in question.

Many different forms are used for the purposes of meditation : sometimes the letters of the Sanscrit or Tibetan alphabets, sometimes the "word of glory", the *pranava* or Aum, sometimes short mystic phrases, the *mantras*, sometimes representations (pictures, statues) of deities. The Tibetans make use also of the incense stick, the red point of which enables them to attain mental concentration rapidly. They make use of "circles of meditation", *Kyilkor*, like the Hindu *mandalas*.

Another series of meditations is concerned with the activity of the mind itself, when in a state of repose or activity. The disciple studies the nature of this interior "force", which is either motionless or in motion, which emerges from and returns to immobility. He notes, finally, the manner in which the mind "apprehends" an object, becomes that object. This process is emphasized in the Tantrik texts, these mental gymnastics which should lead to the disciple "transforming" himself into the object meditated upon.

Finally the student begins to practise "formless" meditation. He begins in the same way, but works with his imagination in such a way as to reduce the mental images perceived. He meditates upon land-scapes which become bare ; upon human beings who are gradually transformed into skeletons. . . . Thus the idea of form is gradually eliminated, then the idea of space, and finally reason merges into an inconceivable "void", which is the intimate and definitive experience of the sole Reality.

CHAPTER VI

CHINESE, JAPANESE AND TIBETAN TECHNIQUES AND THEIR ACCORD WITH THE PRACTICE OF HINDU YOGA

I WROTE at the beginning of this work that Yoga is essentially the basis of all Asiatic mysticism. This chapter, in the course of which we will rapidly compare the various oriental techniques, will support this contention.

CHINESE TRADITION

In the Taoist texts, but most of all in those which have to do with funeral rites, singular analogies with Hindu tradition are to be found.

In the *Annals*—I follow the *Bamboo Chronicle* (*Tchou-chou-ki-nien*)—the idea of survival after death is already quite clearly stated, 3,000 years before Christ. The Chinese Ancients believed that at death man was divided into two parts : *the higher soul* which is subtile, and which rises towards the heights, and *the lower soul*, which is denser, and which goes down into the earth with the corpse. The higher soul is like a smoke, a vapour.

The ritual of *Tcheou*, which belongs to the official ancestral cult of the third dynasty,* states that there

---

* All these fragments are given by Father Leon Wieger in his *History of the Religious Beliefs and Philosophies of China* (Hien-hien, 1927).

were in the Temple seven tablets bearing the names of ancestors. The first of these, placed at the back or middle, was immovable. The six others, arranged in two ranks called *tchao* and *mou*, progressed rank by rank towards the dignity of Ancient, pushed forward by those behind, by the newcomers. When the two ranks of three were complete, and a newcomer had to be given a place, the tablet at the head of the first rank was taken out of the Temple and replaced. It became *t'iao*.

The Emperor honoured his ancestors by libations, oblations, offerings before their tablets. This ceremony took place every three months before each of the seven tablets. Every five years a feast was offered to the seven tablets collectively.

The important thing is that besides the offerings before the tablets, the two souls of the ancestors were evoked—first of all separately. The higher soul was called from the celestial regions by the sound of music, the lower soul from the centre of the earth by the smell of wine spilt as a libation. The ancestors, say the texts, do not eat, but they can smell. Seats were prepared for the evoked dead. The Chinese commentator adds that the gestures were symbolic, the ancestors having no longer the same needs as human beings.

Mong-K'eue or, popularly, *Mong-zeu* (Master Mong), who became known as Mencius (372–289 B.C.), gives some details from the *Seuchou* canons about these two "souls". The higher soul, he says, comes into existence and grows by the absorption and condensation of the subtile matter called median. This subtile matter, informed by the universal norm, is diffused at random.

By means of repeated ordered acts, this confused diffusion becomes a definite instinct of order, of natural knowledge.

The Taoists have always admitted the existence of these two souls ; the higher soul, HOUM or *chenn*, is reincarnated. This reincarnation takes place either in the foetus of a pregnant woman when her time for delivery has come, such foetus having been informed during the pregnancy only with an inferior soul, or in the corpse of a newly dead man or animal. The resurrection of a dead man is quite a natural thing in China. The higher soul can take up its abode at one time or another in the body of a living man. When the higher soul has left the body the lower soul can preserve the latter for a longer or shorter space of time. Then it is extinguished and the body falls into dust. This lower soul corresponds to the subtile body of Hindu philosophy.

When the lower soul, which is not reasonable, is very strong, it preserves the body for a long time and uses it for its own purposes. This body, informed by a lower soul only, is called Kiancheu, and is a frightful vampire, stupid and ferocious. To avoid this misfortune every body which does not decompose normally after death should be burnt. A skeleton, a skull, even a bone, may be informed by a very strong lower soul, which still adheres to it, and may commit, after many centuries, all kinds of evil deeds.*

During dreams the higher soul leaves the body by the great fontanel at the top of the skull, and wanders.

---

* This should be compared with Egyptian tradition concerning the mummy.

The things dreamed are those with which it meets during its strolls. While it is wandering the higher soul may be captured or may lose its way. It can't find its body. When this happens, either the lower soul makes the body continue to live, or the lower soul is affected and the body decomposes.

A story from *T'ai-p'ing Koang-Ki* which is cited by Father Dore* gives a good illustration of this distinction between the two souls. It is as follows :

Nan-tch'ang-hien and *Kiang-Si* were two young men who were studying together and who were bound to each other by a great friendship. One of them died suddenly. The other knew nothing about it. One evening when he had just gone to bed his comrade opened the door, entered and sat down. He said : "It isn't ten days since we parted and behold, I am dead. I am a Koei. But my friendship for you endures. For that reason I have come to say good-bye to you." As fear prevented the other from answering, the dead man continued : "If I had come to injure you would I speak to you in such friendly-wise ? Have no fear. I have come to confide my last wishes to you."

"What do you want ?" asked the live man.

"This . . . My old mother is seventy, my wife is not yet thirty. A few sheaves of corn every year would be enough to support them. Please take charge of them. I have left some good manuscripts. I would ask you to publish them, that some memorial of me may remain. . . . I owe some money to a seller of writing-brushes. I would ask you to pay this debt."

---

* *Research on Chinese Superstitions*, quoted by Father Wieger.

"I will do all that."

"Thank you," said the Koei. "I have nothing more to do here"—and he went out.

The living man recovered from his fright and his affection for his friend awakened. He recalled him. The friend re-entered and sat down again on the edge of the bed. But when the living man looked at him he was quite different, his eyes were fixed, his face disfigured, and there was a stink as of a corpse.

"Go away," cried the living man ; but the dead man didn't stir.

"Go away," repeated the living man, frightened. The dead man rose but did not go away. Terrified, the living man got up from his bed, but the dead one ran after him. He kept behind him the whole time. Finally, worn out, the living man jumped over a wall and fell down on the other side. . . . The dead man couldn't cross the wall, but he tried to spit in the other's face.

Day came. Passers-by found the young man lying on the ground and revived him. They informed the family of the dead man, who sought the corpse which had disappeared. They took it away and buried it.

This singular narrative is thus explained by Chinese commentators : The higher soul is good, the lower soul is wicked. The former is humane, the latter is brutal. The young man was at first visited by the higher, the good soul of his friend. But the lower soul, the physical soul, the corpse-soul (the lower subtile body of Hindu tradition) had followed the higher soul. When the young man recalled the higher soul which had left him, it was the lower soul which

came, that stupid and bestial entity belonging to the
human being. The higher soul of the dead man
treated the living friend as his friend, the lower soul
nearly killed him. All vampires, all wandering corpses,
are lower souls which have become incorporated.
Only a man who has reached the point of perfection
(a yogi one might say) can make the lower soul good.
This rarely happens. . . .

We will now state as exactly as possible the qualities
of these two "souls"; the *Sing-li ta-ts'uan* of the
Ming dynasty gives us some interesting particulars.

There are two states of matter: *koei* (−) and *chenn* (+);
koei is the apogee of the state *yinn*, *chenn* is the apogee
of the state *yang*. If we contemplate evolving matter,
its progression is *chenn* (positive), its regression is
koei (negative); but the progression already contains
the germ of future regression and vice versa.

The two souls, *hounn* and *p'ai* are "material" (they
are manifestations). The *hounn*—the higher soul—is
hot, is the energy of the breath, the centre of the
intelligence. The *p'ai*—the lower soul—is cold. It
is the energy of the sperm, the centre of memory. The
union of the *hounn* and the *p'ai* is necessary to life.
Their separation causes death. At the beginning of
all things the first union of *Yinn* and *Yang* produced
water, which is the universal *p'ai*. Hence a cold *p'ai*
is first produced, to which a hot *hounn* is attached by
the action of respiration. The *p'ai* precedes, the *hounn*
follows.

We must not distinguish between two matters, but
between two aspects of the same matter which are

differentiated, which oppose one another in the *Yinn* and the *Yang*, the one passive and regressive, the other active and progressive. During progression—the Chinese call it the *yang* time—the *p'ai* obeys, the *houun* commands. During regression—*yinn* time—the *p'ai* commands, the *houun* obeys.

The *houun* is the quintessence of *yang*, it synthetizes the faculties of the human body. The *p'ai* is the quintessence of *yinn* and synthetizes the bodily form.

Man, having been made, naturally comes to an end. The *houun* rises towards heaven, the *p'ai* descends towards the earth, for the hot rises and the cold falls. Birth is followed by death, the end follows the beginning.

The *houun* and the *p'ai*, as we have seen, are both material. They are made of subtile matter ; the *p'ai* is inert, the *houun* is active. Ghosts that haunt and otherwise make disturbances are *houun* which are not yet dissipated, because, separated before their time, they were not "ripe". In that condition they can do these things. They are, provisionally, in Nature what lumps are in dough, that disappear in the course of kneading. Everything evolves. Nothing lasts. Since the beginning and all through time, all beings have been *yinn* and *yang*, regression and progression.

In a waking state, *yang*, the *p'ai* is absorbed by the *houun*, which, coming out through the eyes and ears, acquires new and exact knowledge. In sleep, *yinn*, the *houun*, which has retired into the *p'ai*, has only a confused memory of former impressions.

Pao-p'ou-tzeyeu or *Keue-houng* (the Master loving simplicity) wrote one of the chief Chinese Taoist works.

This was a Master who approximated in an extraordinary degree to Hindu yogis, in the curious details
which he gives of the transformation of the human
body by means of certain exercises. These mysterious
processes made it possible for men to become terrestrial
Genies, we might say "liberated men".

These terrestrial Genies wander on celebrated
mountains, the great mountain chain of *k'oum-lunn* ;
others retire into the mountains and wear their
"former body", the body of an old man as a rule,
often ugly and deformed, with hair and nails untended.

The means prescribed by *Keue-houng* for becoming a
Genie are yoga. Father Wieger (loc. cit.) gives an
excellent summary of them, which I follow :

(1) *Assimilation of air*. Air should be breathed in
through the nostrils slowly, so gently that no intake
of the breath should be perceptible, and it should stop
when the thorax begins to be dilated. Then the breath
should be held as long as possible, at least for the time
in which one counts from *one to a hundred and twenty*.
Afterwards it should be breathed out through the
mouth, completely, and so gently that a swan's feather
hung before the face should not move. Then there
should be inhalation again, expiration, and so on.

The theoretical aim of this process, according to
Keue-houng, is a return to the respiration of the fœtus
in the womb, by which the embryo grows continually,
giving off nothing. The ideal would be to hold in the
air for the time it takes to count from *one* to *a thousand*,
for the air restores and vivifies the body.

The air must be living *yang* and not dead *yinn*.
This exercise should be done between midnight and

noon. During this period the air is *yang*. From noon until midnight it is *yinn*.

Those who do breathing exercises should be vegetarians. Besides the renovation of the organism, says the Chinese author, this exercise tends to perfect abstraction, and in consequence perfect concentration of the mind. It gives the body health and absolute peace.

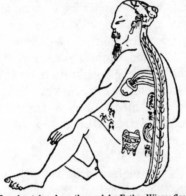

Engraving of a *Tao-chen* taken from the work by Father Wieger (loc. cit.). It is a very curious system of Chinese Yoga. The vertebral column and the chief nâdîs are clearly marked. The secondary chakra of the heart is connected with the vertebral column, as is also the chakra of the stomach.
    The stove is "the matrix of transcendent being"; it is remarkable that its place is approximately that of kundalini in the Hindu texts.

(2) *Management of the sperm*. *Keue-houng* declares in the first instance that these exercises should be taught orally. These are Tantrik practices which are found in certain schools in India, and which act upon the sexual energy. This may be taken as a new proof either of an exchange of traditional doctrine between China and India, or of the existence of an immemorial tradition.

(3) *Ingestion of the drug of immortality*. Here we

find the principles which have guided Eastern and Western alchemy. This alchemy is not only physical and material. It acts also on subtile matter.

Keue-houng quotes several Taoist Masters, *tao-cheu*, who lived like yogis, without nourishment for two or three years. He relates that King Kind of Ou (258–263) placed the *tao-cheu Cheu-tch'ounn* in a cage for more than a year, and that he lived on just a little water.

To sum up, without entering into detail as regards certain practices of Chinese Yoga, we may state that there is a profound similitude between the doctrines of Hindu Yoga and Chinese Taoism. This identity does not result from the possibility of cultural exchange alone, but also from a unanimous tradition concerning the exercises and meditations necessary in order to open the subtile Centres of Energy in the human body.

. .

JAPANESE TRADITION

It is chiefly the *Shingon* and *Zen* schools which yield interesting texts. These two schools are essentially mystic and the meditations which they use are similar to the teachings of Yoga. On the Japanese *mandala* (*himitsu*) we find the letters of the Sanscrit alphabet. The contact between the Japanese and Hindu schools of Yoga is thus actually proved.

The *Shingon* (the word means *True Word*) declares * that all activities in the world are only varied aspects of the essence of the universe. The EGO which is in man and in things expresses itself outwardly. We must

---

* See the excellent work on *Buddhist Sects in Japan*, by Steinilber-Oberlin and Kuni Matsuo (Paris : G. Cres, 1930).

conform the rhythm of our life to the great activities of Heaven.

Shingon teaching is given under two forms : Exoteric (ken-kyo) and esoteric (mitsou-kyo). The school makes use of circles of meditation (himitsu mandara), graphic and symbolic, which represent the universe. Mystic letters (the letters of the Sanscrit alphabet) are put in certain places to concentrate the psychic force which issues from the representation. The relationship of these mandalas with the Tibetan meditation pictures is remarkable.

The basis of the Shingon cult is the realization of the profound unity between the deity and the worshipper, which is the basis of Hindu Yoga as we have seen. A mystic ritual is thus used in which the sound and the secret sign of the deity worshipped are largely used.

The Zen school (from *zenna*, which means *dhyâna* (contemplation) is Taoist and Chinese in origin, and reckons among its spiritual patriarchs the celebrated Bodhidharma, who lived in the sixth century of our era. According to this school, Nature does more than explain itself, it suggests in us that we should understand ourselves. It is a monastic school, extremely simple and harsh. Its discipline is severe and strict. The Zen methods of meditation in the zendo (the Hall of Meditation) in the depths of Mokugio, are very special.

The base of Zen is the slowing down of satori (Chinese Wu), mental relaxation, intuitive contemplation of the deep nature of things. Mental relaxation is not brought about by logical reasoning, but rather by an emotional and spiritual shock, the consciousness is plunged into the Beyond of the mind, by an interior spiritual emotion. "You have found yourselves at last" a Zen Master will say to his disciples.

Zen is, in its processes of meditation, in its methods, in its cosmic conception, in all points similar to Hindu Yoga, of which it is the spiritual son, through the Hindu missionaries who came to China. Breath control forms a part of the Zen exercises. Mental concentration (sesshin) is habitual in the zendo.

TIBETAN TRADITION

I can only outline here the mystic processes of Tibet, which excellent works have to a great extent popularized in France. But I may assert the close and deep union between the Tibetan technique of meditation and Hindu Yoga. The one owes everything to the other, since the Hindu Tantrik missionaries introduced the lamaic cult into Tibet. The learned lamas who came from India, such as Marpa, only conveyed and translated the Hindu Tantrik texts.

It is known that in Tibet, besides the lamaic organizations, the yellow caps (Gelong-pa), and the red caps (Khagyud-pa), there are adepts "of the direct way", the Naldjorpas. They live in caves and hermitages, lost in the mountains, and sometimes even isolate themselves in Tsham khang (from Tsham, meaning solitude).

One of the rules of their yoga is that "the breath is the steed of the mind, which is the rider". The regularization of the breath to calm the mind is thus one of their chief preoccupations. It is useless to give

details of their methods.   They are exactly the same
as those which I have already given, since the texts and
oral tradition are identical.   The words alone differ.

One finds in Tibet the circles of meditation or
Kyilkhor, diagrams, sometimes very large, traced on
the earth with powder of different colours; and orna-
mented with incense sticks, representations of deities
(*Torma*), made of dough, etc.   These diagrams are
given by the Master to his disciples as a *ten*, that which
concentrates the mind and in which the manas should
sink itself, with which it should identify itself.

Deities—symbolizing the forces of the cosmos and
of the human being—"come out of" and "re-enter" the
kyilkhor and the body of the person meditating.   There
is a constant and living communion between the disciple and his mental creation.   Sometimes the whole
kyilkhor reduces itself to a single point and *enters*
into the body of the person meditating and is re-
absorbed in him, entering between the two eyebrows.

The disciple thus learns to "become" the object and
to realize the creative power of the mind.   Some yogis
are even able to create, by the power of the mind,
complete beings, living gods, personalities (the *Ydam*)
which they are afterwards to dissolve.   They realize
in very truth the illusory nature of all things.

CHAPTER VII

THE SEXUAL PROBLEM IN YOGA AND TANTRISM

YOGA which has studied the human being in his most secret manifestations has not forgotten the most mysterious force in man : the sexual force.

In a preceding work* I wrote as follows concerning the Tantrik notion of the sexual mystery :

"How many errors are still current in the West on this subject ! Who has not read the adjectives 'shameful and repugnant' applied to the cult either of the *lingam* or of the divine *Shaktis* ? But now European psychology has begun to penetrate into the mysteries of the human subconscious mind, and to discover there the primary importance of the sexual power. Freud has accustomed the philosophers to look the problem in the face. Tantrik initiates studied the problem long ago in detail. Must they be reproached for having sounded one of the great mysteries of the human being ? Their technical books on this subject are extremely precise, and it may be that some passages, badly translated but above all badly commentated, may have frightened the well-known modesty of the West. What would we say if some of Freud's pages were thus translated and interpreted ? Would we not justly accuse the translator or com-

---

* *Secret India and Its Magic* (Les Œuvres Françaises, Paris, 1937).

mentator of bad faith, voluntary or involuntary ?
The Hindu Tantriks, wiser yet, preferred to keep
silence and shrug their shoulders, but this attitude
renders yet more difficult the approach to these books
and to their qualified interpreters.

"I will say simply that when Freud made of the *libido*
an independent force, which has not *necessarily* a
sexual goal, he is in absolute agreement with Tantrik
doctrine. This force may be displaced in one direction
or another. Desire does not necessarily manifest
itself in the sexual act. It transforms itself, disguises
itself, in a way hides itself. . . . This force is, in
itself, like the tension of the bow, which knows not
whither the arrow will go. This 'tension' may relax
in the sublime activities of art, religion, music, prayer ;
it may also take paths that are obscure, twisting and
fatal. The *libido* itself, without a definite form,
without an aim, may manifest itself in good or evil,
like the *dardje* of Tibet, the Tantric weapon *par ex-
cellence*, which turns to the right or the left according
to the will of the wielder.

"Nietzsche has said that the field of activity of
sexuality in the human being attains the highest peaks
of his mind. The Tantriks have never said otherwise.
But instead of looking down and declaring that the
problem is untouchable and 'disgusting' they have
expressed and noted the various manifestations of the
force which leads the world.

"For the problem remains the same and, unconsciously, the ardent search for happiness is the interior,
truncated, often unhappy expression of the interior
force which *wills* the expansion of the human being

into the divine. By all means man wishes to expand his consciousness : by dogmas, by love, by prayer, by magic, he would fain attain the 'beyond' of consciousness, that beatitude which is no longer human. Primitive sexual rites are a means to making this state of consciousness emerge. Drugs are another. The fact remains that the sexual act is the most powerful of levers—one which shakes human power to its depths. In this book, which is not a medical book, I will not give details of the processes used to set in action the slumbering forces of the human being. I will simply say that a subject of this kind is approached in the Tantrik schools with fear and reverence. Hindu wisdom respects the most direct representation, the most concrete, and the most efficacious of the divine on earth. We have here to do with one of the major mysteries.

"In the West it is difficult to study this problem. Deep and complex currents of inferiority complex have flowed on for a long time, and love has been either shamed or dreaded, hidden or exalted. Violent reactions have succeeded profound revulsions.

"Tantrism teaches that the vital force kundalini has its corresponding force on the nervous and physical planes, the force of the sexual organs. Tantrik Hatha Yoga strives to regulate this force by will and mental discipline, it tries to sublimate the developed force and thus to awaken the subtle centres. We have already said a few words on the subject.

"This awakening of the sexual force takes place with the wife—the *Shakti* of the Tantriks. But I met a **Tantrik who lived alone and who showed me his** sacred trident. 'That is my wife,' said he. One makes contact here with complex and difficult rites which cannot be summarized without being distorted.

"Whilst the finest mystic chants, both Christian and Musulman, are in the form of love poems, the Tantrik texts, Hindu and Tibetan, use sexual comparisons to reinforce their images and their doctrine. Thus method, the will, are solar and male (it is the Tibetan *gab*) ; wisdom, imagination are lunar and feminine (Tibetan *youm*). There must be a union between the two, a union as close and as ardent as the sexual union, for complete realization.

"The Yoga rites contain a profound doctrine ; it may be summarized thus : 'Identification of the wife with the divine Shakti.' It must be understood that Asia has never looked upon the sexual act from the point of view of 'morality' dear to our modest contemporaries. For Asia incapacity is a weakness and not a virtue. If a man wishes to live in continence, and thus sublimate (consciously or not) his sexual force in mental energies, he is at liberty to do so. But he is not above the married man who follows the natural law.

"As regards this latter, the Tantrik rites permit him to identify his wife (and inversely the husband for the woman becomes the god) with the divine Shakti, the goddess. The act of love thus becomes an act of worship in intense joy.

"This path, if mental discipline is strictly maintained, leads to a spiritual realization which is possible in marriage. But I believe that the heavy psychic atavism which rules in the West renders this way dangerous in view of possible deviations.

"It is easy to guess what these deviations might be : the use of the sexual force for spiritual vampirism or for the ends of black magic. These rites exist in Asia and the Voodoo is their counterpart among the negroes. Without entering into details, I will simply say—for the benefit of imprudent experimenters—that all women are not usable for such rites, but there must be special signs when they are chosen, and inversely. These rites are dangerous and useless for spiritual realization. I will recall a phrase of a Hindu Mahatma : 'Blind and mad is the man who, prejudicing his mental power, derogates from the moral laws which the Sages have laid down.' "

CHAPTER VIII

DEATH, THE STATES AFTER DEATH AND
REINCARNATION ACCORDING TO YOGA

THE moral laws which Western religious forms maintained up to our days extended beyond death. In the social state in which we were for a long time, severe and pitiless physical punishments ordained by the social codes were continued naturally into the other world. The West has always been afraid of death, and is so still.

Asia has a quite different idea of this problem. Death is for it just a change in the human complex, and the Eastern is disquieted not about the fact of dying, but about the need to be reincarnated, that is to say to return into the "Wheel of the World", and to suffer in the world again. It is the suppression of suffering that is the basis of the Asiatic methods of liberation. The wisdom of Asia does not stop at a transformation of man, but it wishes to liberate the human being from the claws of pain.

Death for the Yoga is an experience, lived through and controlled. When I mentioned this problem in Asia I always heard from those I addressed the same answer: "I have seen, I know. . . ." It is a heard experience, a direct testimony which I have often had the privilege of receiving. The doors of death open before the living man who is free from fear and from the desire to live.

In order to understand the mechanism of death we must keep well in mind the composition of the human being as we have studied it in the preceding pages. In him, in his living state, the whole universe is present ; the four kingdoms of living creatures ; fire, air, water and earth are under his domination which represents symbolically the Tibetan dordje with four points, that sceptre of universal domination.

Yoga teaches first of all that certain dramatic phenomena which accompany the death agony are somewhat like epileptic fits, in which the human being shouts, rolls, seems to suffer terribly, and yet is absolutely unconscious of his state, the only thing he feels being great fatigue.

The phenomenon of death is caused by the profound disturbance of the circulation of the prâna in the nâdîs. Illness, physical and nervous exhaustion have their effect in course of time on the subtile bodies. It is they which decide the issue of life or death, except, of course, in the case of an accident.

So as to prevent the prâna and the subtile bodies separating from the dying in a wrong way, the Tantrik rites direct that the dying man should be turned on to his right side and that the jugular veins on each side of the neck should be moderately pressed. It seems that when this is done the blood brought by the arteries remains longer in the brain instead of spreading to the abdominal cavity as happens usually at death.

Yoga asserts that the prânic fluid goes towards the navel, where there is a secondary subtile centre ; thence during the death agony it rises towards the heart. The *manas*, the mind, also tends from the brain towards the heart, and the union of these two currents in the centre of the heart forms a subtile entity which disengages itself by degrees from the breast of the dying man, and commences to "be" on the subtile plane, which is that of its heavier "matter", the matter of the physical body only existing as a support.

But Yoga teaches that this disengagement or separation profoundly disturbs the human being who thus duplicates himself, and hinders the phenomena of spiritual realization taking place in the way we have just seen. It is necessary that the subtile forces and the *manas* which contains the consciousness of the dying man should come out of the top of the head through a fissure called Brahma's hole, which plays a great part in Asiatic anatomy.

If the human being disengages himself thus, says the tradition, he retains a clear consciousness of his state, and, above all, at a given moment (twenty to twenty-five minutes after apparent death), experiences an ecstatic state which is an absolute reproduction of the *Samâdhi* of the yogi, a state which permits him to realize his union with the divine. This is an opportunity open to every human being who dies, but unfortunately very few become aware of this possibility.

The sensations of a dying man are various, and depend on his mental and moral state. The material elements are dissolving in him, and at each dissolution a new sensation is experienced by the dying man.

There is the physical sensation of *pressure* which comes with the loss of control of the facial muscles when the element *earth* disappears into the element *water*.

There is the physical sensation of *intense cold*, then of *heat* and the loss of hearing, when the element *water* disappears into the element *fire*.

There is a physical sensation of corporeal *explosion* and of dissolution accompanied by loss of sight when the element *fire* disappears into the element *air*.

The dying man, before falling into a deep sleep, then experiences this vision—often fugitive—of the complete realization of which we have spoken ; but if he is not a yogi or a saint, if desires attach him to the "Wheel of the World", he turns away from this "luminous void" which offends his personality.

Then come the states after death which, in principle, are the reactions of desires and mental forms on their generator. The disembodied soul is no longer protected by the strong envelope of the flesh and is living on a plane where all thought has its form, where every desire becomes a reality. He has acquired the habit of continually generating thoughts, and making his consciousness tend towards the realization of certain desires. He can do this no more. The intensity of his exasperated desires, which are bound to disappear, give rise to an educative suffering, just and real.

The Tantrik texts, absolutely identical with the Egyptian texts, have symbolized these sufferings, these post-mortem experiences by forces with human heads or animals which have issued from the body of the discarnate and which react upon him with a violence corresponding to the generative power. These are the

dramas of judgment, of purgatory. The literature of
experimental psychics has given us numerous docu-
ments concerning these post-mortem dramas, and in
them one can see how strong the impression of these
dramas is on the minds of those who experience them.*
Post-mortem evolution tends to convince the discarnate of the unreality of the physical and subtle
world.

Very often the violent desires of the discarnate and
the law of *Karma* ordaining retribution for past acts
does not permit of this liberation or this awakening.
The human being has the fruit, sweet or bitter, of his
past existence, and of the profound tendencies of his
being, such as he has made it. Thus there are places
of peace and of joy (the paradise of the various re-
ligions) or of suffering and pain (the purgatories and
hells). But the Yoga asserts that retribution is in
exact proportion to the crimes and the faults com-
mitted, and that what we have to do with is the
exhaustion of a mental force generated by the human
being in his ignorance. Knowledge alone liberates man.

---

* The contradictory descriptions given at séances are explained
by the fact that the discarnate lives in the world he mentally creates,
and of which he cannot get rid. I only know a few cases of experimenters which confirm the Asiatic teaching. We recommend, for
instance, for reading the mediumistic messages of Albert Pouchard
in *The Other World and its Infinite Possibilities* (Geneva, 1936). This
recognizes, for the first time in my experience, the complete sub-
jectivity of the creations and the world which he meets in his
experiences after death.

The translation of *Bar-do thos' grol*, edited by Dr. Evans-Wentz in
English and published in France by Maisonneuve, is also to be
recommended. In it we find the same traditions concerning the
states after death, currents of Tantrism originating in India which
have penetrated deeply into Tibet and superimposed themselves on
the conceptions of the primitive society of Central Asia.

In accordance with their Karma the discarnate, the *preta*, live a pleasant or painful life, either in stupid indifference or amid the dramas which attach it, by reason of unsatisfied desire, to the places which they "haunt", as the cant expression goes.

Little by little, however, desire is exhausted, a "second death" (judgment before the "Lords of Death", according to Asiatic tradition) takes place. It corresponds with the dissolution of the subtile bodies, formed by the "desire to be", which were the temporary envelope of the human being. Just as the material body returns to the bosom of nature and serves again to make the physical supports of life (vegetable, animal and human), so the subtile bodies dissolve into the planes of matter corresponding to them, to which, however, they impart a very strong impregnation (a smell as a yogi said to me) proceeding from the being whose envelope they were.

When a human being is formed again these subtile elements return to him in accordance with the Karma law of affinity, and sometimes bring with them contrary tendencies, contradictory urges, diverse personalities in the same human being. Then the belief arises that there are memories of past reincarnations, while in reality the problem is more complex. That which is reincarnated or transmigrated is the higher element of the human being, which has not been able to escape the "Wheel of the World".

Then the drama of reincarnation is played. The desires in germ of his Karma tend to lead the human being back towards the same plane. According to Yoga, it must be clearly stated, only the flow of life rises and falls, disincarnates and reincarnates itself. The Ego is a spectator, it "shadows" as the Tibetans say, the temporary human constituent, it does not incorporate itself in it—any more than the Ocean can "enter" into a wave.

Hence to believe that one becomes an animal or a plant is a mistake, just as it is a mistake to believe in a *static condition* after death in an eternal paradise or hell.   In reality the human constituent is very complex. Its heavy and coarse elements may descend and become animal.   It is, taking it altogether, a question of the quality of vibrations.   Other elements may, by the law of like to like, animate vegetable and primitive forms.   Inversely sufficiently evolved animal and vegetable forms incorporate themselves in a "human constituent" and form those "animal" types, often very curious, which one meets among humans.   Asiatics explain thus the fœtus or human monsters with the head or body of animals which are much more frequent than one would believe.

We, in our turn, colour the whole of nature.   Our rule over the universe is real and effective.   The subtile waves go and come in slow or rapid evolution, and rule the complex laws of Karma : the living communion between all the elements of the Cosmos.

CHAPTER IX

THE PRACTICE OF YOGA IN THE WEST—THE MESSAGE OF ASIA

THE question of the possibilities for Yoga in the West has been frequently discussed ; but either the translated texts gave such a complexity of methods of meditation, the terms used are so strange, that the Western student, with the best will in the world, feels lost in the atmosphere that is incomprehensible for him. Or perhaps, again, attempts to popularize give him a "Westernized Yoga", a simple manual of physical gymnastics without any connection with the admirable texts which they pretend to popularize.

One should know how to extract without destroying and to adapt without distorting. The deities, the descriptions of the Tantric *mandalas*, the classifications of human forces, are, according to the Asiatic texts, essentially symbolical. They represent energies, planes of the universe, and can thus be perfectly understood and realized by either an Oriental or an Occidental.

It is obvious that certain technical terms must be retained, for our science of man has no equivalent word —but this can be easily done, and I have endeavoured here not to overcharge my text with useless Sanscrit words. An index at the end of this volume will enable the reader to find out the meaning of the Asiatic words used.

This having been settled, it is easy to see that the great bases of Yoga are simple ideas. A Western can understand Yoga perfectly—his own yoga—if he reflects on the great laws given in the course of this book. He should know, besides, that he has in himself a living and faithful light, an incomparable instructor who only waits to be listened to. But we must know how to listen. . . .

Who cannot practise suppressing ignorance, selfishness and desire ? The company of the Sages, holy books, texts concerning illumination, may be found all around. If one would read explanations of the great Asiatic treatises on Consciousness and the Ego there are excellent translations of the authentic texts.

The basis has still to be laid of a certain discipline (postures and rhythmic breathing), accompanied by mental discipline. The essential elements of this discipline have been given here, it suffices to practise them and to create the new "habits" indispensable to the new automatisms which one wishes to establish in oneself.

There remains the serious problem of religion. It is not necessary to forsake the religion to which one belongs, but fear must be suppressed—that psychical and spiritual poison which does so much damage.

It is essential to realize that a sincere religious aspiration invariably leads to a spiritual realization. It should also be understood that dogma is the *exterior bark* of personal experience, which, only, can be individual and profound. One may very well get great consolation and unforgettable spiritual illumination in a church where the rites, the people and the gestures shock one.

Yoga teaches that the great spiritual currents are of the cosmic order and absolutely universal. It is just that the mind colours the spiritual vision. The habit of straining one's will and attention creates gleaming mental forms which, in their turn, help the disciple. Let us never forget, either, that the communion of the wise is a reality, not material as some have said, but very strong on the subtile planes. The fact of directing one's attention towards them gives rise to a contact, almost automatic, with beings who help, who protect and who are called Masters.

It is this patient, profound research into oneself, one's Ego (the Hindu Atmâ) which is the key to the cult that sustains and animates. The Ego remains. IT alone is eternal.

The realization of the Supreme Identity is the goal. It is liberation from the currents of life, the troubled inflows, the incessant transmigrations that is the object. Not that "life" is an accursed thing, to be cast away. That is a barbarous, a primitive idea. But the aim of man is to co-operate with the Divine, and to be its instrument in matter. It is through him—and only through him—that the great plan of Brahma can be realized and his work of love finished. Man, like a great brazier, purifies and transforms the cosmos. Through him flow the undeveloped currents, the heavy "lumps" of earth, impregnated with animality. And man transforms them, purifies them, balances them. He is like Fire, he transmutes and dissolves the coarse elements into radiant light, into beneficent warmth. With him, thanks to him, all Nature is raised. The

Master kneads the rebellious dough of the world. He alone transforms the world.

The message of Asia through Yoga is the liberation of man. As a sage said to me in India : "Death follows life and life prepares the way for death. Such is the Law. . . . But do not fix thine attention on the changing things of life, on the births, the deaths, the sufferings of beings. Transport thy gaze to That which directs and leads the wheel, to Him Who is *responsible for all things*. He is within thee, he awaits thee. . . . But do not believe that *That* is defined and that thy mind can easily grasp it. There must be a deep peace, an acute clairvoyance beyond all personal consciousness.

"Faults give rise to acts, and acts, again, generate acts, sooner or later. The wheel must be stopped, the past must be exhausted, the other road must be taken. All men seek happiness, and their mistake lies in seeking wrongly that peace, that liberty which they believe they will derive from the things of the world and which is a new chain. The search for liberty is the first instinctive act of man when he awakens to the divine. And when he realizes his Ego, the Divine residing in him, he is free. . . .

"How then can the law of Karma be valid for him? He is detached from his own acts, by his knowledge he avoids new bonds, and his union with the divine, with his EGO, puts him on a plane of deliverance. Life has become for him a deep harmony, an admirable edifice of the Divine, and death is the gentle hand of Kâli, that tranforms, purifies and lifts up. . . ."

INDEX OF SANSCRIT WORDS

NOTE.—In the transcription of Sanscrit words it was impossible for typographical reasons to use the scientific transcription, with the points underneath for the linguals and accents for certain gutturals and palatals. It will, however, be easy for specialists to reconstruct the correct Sanscrit word.

The index which follows gives the meanings of the words used.

I have used the order of the European alphabet in order to facilitate search. (Note that *u* is pronounced *oo*, and *c, tch*.)

A

Advaitavâdi. A yoga state in which the duality of the world disappears.

Agni. The god of Fire ; the animating heat which resides in every living being ; the internal fire.

Ahamkâra. The sense of INDIVIDUALITY.

Ajnâ chakra. The subtile centre situated between the two eyebrows.

Akasha. The principle of the fifth material element, Ether.

Alambusha. Name of a nâdî.

Ananda. Beatitude.

Ananda Kanda. Secondary chakra at the place of the heart.

Ap. The material element in water.

Arddha nârishvara. The god Shiva in his androgynous form.

Arjana. A Hindu prince whose dialogue with Krishna on the eve of the great war of Kurukshetra forms the subject of the songs of the Gita.

Asana. The postures of the body taught by Yoga.

Atmâ. The supreme EGOm Brahma acting through the human being.

B

Bhagavad Gitâ. The song of the Blessed One, one of the classic texts of India.

Bhâkti yoga. The yoga of devotion.

Bhûtas. The five elements of matter.

Bhrûmadhya-drishti. Prolonged staring at the tip of the nose.

Bîja. The notion of the root, the germ, peculiar to Tantrism, which resolves manifestation into a series of bîjas which have themselves issued from the generator.

Bindu. A dot, word by word ; that is, a centre of creative energy.

Bodhini. One of the Shakti of subtile manifestation in the causal plane.

Brahma. The universal and impersonal Principle ; THE EGO in one's self.

Brahmarandra. The lotus with a thousand petals situated above the head.

Brahmanâdî. The royal road, the very delicate nâdî situated at the centre of the sushumnâ, in the interior of the cerebro-spinal axis.

Buddhi. The ray emanating from the EGO and illuminating the individual state.

C

Chintâmanistava. Text of Shankaracharya.

Chit. The universal consciousness of the EGO from the point of view of its relation with its sole object, Beatitude.

Chitrini. One of the nâdîs situated at the interior of the cerebro-spinal axis.

Cid-anu. Atom of consciousness ; one of the aspects of the creative consciousness.

Citta. State of mind passing rapidly from one object to another without reason for doing so.

D

Dâkini. The presiding deity of the first chakra ; muladhara.

Damaru. The drum peculiar to the Tantrik rites, sometimes made of two human skulls cut in half and fixed together at the top and suspended on straps of leather.

Dhârana. The concentration of the mind on an object.

Dhyâna. A state of contemplation arrived at by concentrating the mind.

G

Gândhâri. One of the secondary nâdîs.

Gange. The sacred river in the north of India ; its symbolism is important.

Garuda. The vehicle of Vishnu, a symbolical animal having the form of a bird.

Gunas. The conditions of universal existence ; its forms of manifestation.

Guru. The spiritual instructor, the Master.

H

Hâkini. The deity who presides over the ajna chakra.

Hamsa. The divine swan, the "vehicle" of Brahma.

Hari-Vishnu. The form of universal energy under its generative and creative aspect.

Hastijivâ. One of the secondary nâdîs.

Hatha Yoga. Yoga based on the purification of the physical body by physical proceedings, postures, respiration, asceticism, etc.

I

Idâ. One of the three principal nâdîs in the human body.

Indriyas. Faculties of sensation and perception in the human body.

Isha. The god who presides over the anahata chakra, at the height of the heart.

Ishwara. "Personality", the supreme principle, both acting and manifesting itself.

J

Jîva. The manifestation of the Ego in jîva is jivâtma, the living human soul.

Jivâtma. The individual manifestation, transitory and contingent to one's self.

Jnâna. Wisdom, traditional consciousness, realized by the intellectual intuition.

Jnâna Yoga. The yoga based on consciousness.

K

Kâkini. The deity who dwells in the anahata chakra, at the height of the heart.

Kali. The Siva aspect, transformative and defensive, of the divine manifestation.

Kalpanâ-matram. The universe as the creation of the mind.

Kanda. A subtile junction where the nâdîs of the body end.

Karanashartra. The causal body of the human being.

Karma. The action, the act and its results.

Karma Yoga. The yoga based on the strict accomplishment of the actions conformable to the social and moral duties.

Kâshi. Name of Benares.

Klim. A Tantrik mantra very much used in rituals.

Kroshna. One of the divine descents or incarnations. His teaching to Arjuna is the subject of the Bhagavad Gita.

Kuhû. One of the secondary nâdîs.

Kumbhaka. The stoppage of the breath between inspiration and expiration.

Kundalini. The divine energy, the cosmic power drowsy and latent in the chakra Muladhara and which is awakened by yoga.

Kurukshetra. The field of battle where Krishna taught Arjana.

L

Lâkini. The deity which resides in the manipura chakra at the height of the navel.

Lakshmi. The joyous and "feminine" aspect of the Divine Wisdom.

Lalanâ chakra. A minor chakra at the base of the palate.

Laya Yoga. A special yoga based on the concentration of the mind on the human interior.

Lingam. The representation of the male generative force in its creative and Shivaesque aspect.

Linga sharira. The totality of the subtile bodies, of the bodies of fire which animate the physical body.

M

Makara. A symbolic monster which supports a letter in the genital chakra.

Manas. The mind, one of the faculties of sensation and action.

Manas Chakra. One of the minor chakras localized in the head.

Mandala. Representations, generally circular, symbols of the cosmic and human forces.

Mani. Means jewel.

Manipûra chakra. A centre of force situated at the height of the navel.

Manomaya Kosha. The mental body.

Mantra. An assemblage of letters the sound of which awakens certain interior forces.

Mantra Yoga. Yoga based on the repetition of these living formulas, which thus act on the human being.

Mâyâ. Illusion, the reflection of the EGO in exterior manifestations which thus appear separate and distinct.

Merudanda. Name of the cerebro-spinal axis.

Moksha. The liberation of the human being by his identification with atma.

Mudrâs. Gestures of the hands which accompany the ritual.

Mukti. Another name for Moksha, deliverance or liberation.

Muktatriveni. The triple knot made by the three principal nâdîs near the chakra of the forehead.

Mûlâdhâra. The chakra placed at the base of the great nâdî and the place where kundalini reposes.

N

Nâda. The human interior sound.

Nâsâgra-drishthi. Prolonged staring at the tip of the nose.

Nirvâna. The extinction of agitation ; serenity ; the state of a being who is subject to no more change or modification.

O

OM. A sacred monosyllable symbolizing the Manifestation of Brahma.

P

Padma. Lotus. The symbolic name of the chakras.

Padmâsana. Posture of the body in the form of a lotus.

Parashakti. The prefix *para* signifies supreme ; the supreme shakti, kundalini.

Parasharira. The causal human body.

Paramâtmâ. The supreme Ego, the universal Spirit.

Patanjali. The codificator of the yoga sutras.

Payasvini. A secondary nâdî.

Pingalâ. One of the three principal nâdîs.

Prakâsha. Luminous ; this word is used to describe states of matter.

Prakriti. The primordial undifferentiated substance, the passive principle, feminine ; producing nature.

Prâna. Vital breath, essence, the subtile energy which circulates in the subtile bodies through the nâdîs.

Prânamaya Kosha. The subtile envelope of the human body which is nearest to the material elements.

Prânâyâma. The sum of the breathing exercises which are intended to regularize the circulation of the prana.

Prayoga. A kind of sexual yoga.

Preta. The discarnate.

Pretya bhava. Transmigration or rebirth.

Prithivi. Terrestrial prana or the essence of the element of earth.

Pûruka. The inhalation of air.

Purusha. Brahma considered as the Supreme Orderer of the human being in whom he dwells, the animator of life.

Pûshâ. One of the secondary nâdîs.

R

Râga. Desire.

Rajas. Name of one of the Gunas.

Rajayoga. The royal yoga, based on essentially mental methods.

Râkini. The deity dominating the genital chakra.

Ram. The ram, the vehicle of Agni, god of Fire.

Râma. Son of Dasharatha, the hero of Ramayana.
Rechakra. The exhalation of the breath.
Rudra. The deity or chakra of the navel.

S

Sâdhu-sanga. The company of the Sages, necessary for the practice of yoga.
Saguna. Meditation *with* form.
Samâdhi. Ecstasy, the union, or rather the identification of the human Ego with the divine EGO.
Samani. One of the causal planes of realization.
Samtosa. The waves of desire.
Sankhini. One of the secondary nâdîs.
Saraswati. Name of one of the sacred rivers of India.
Saraswati. Name of a secondary nâdî.
Sat. Pure being.
Sattwa. One of the three Gunas.
Savasana. One of the postures of yoga, called the pose of death.
Shâkini. The deity presiding over the centre of the throat.
Shakti. Productive will, generating divine aspects; the feminine and passive aspect of the divine formative activity.
Shama. Calm, tranquillity of the senses.
Shiva. One of the three aspects of Brahma, showing his activity as transforming and purifying.
Shivalinga. The creative, generative power of Brahma.
Shodhana. The purification of the nâdîs.
Shûnya. The great void, the supreme light.
Soma chakra. A minor chakra in the head.
Sthûla sharira. The material human body.
Sukhsohmasharira. The subtile human body.
Sushumna. One of the principal nâdîs.
Sushupta sthana. The state of deep sleep.
Svâdhishthâna. The chakra of the genital centre.

Svapna Sthana. Dream state.
Svastika. The ancient symbol of fire.
Svayambhu. Another name for Shivalinga.

T

Taijâsa. The luminous ; the condition of the human being in the state of dream or the discarnate state.
Tamas. One of the three Gunas ; a descending force, a force of inertia.
Tanmâtras. The elementary essences of the five human senses.
Tâpa. Burning ; the state of matter called free.
Tattwas. The subtile energies ; 25 in manifestation.
Têjas. The essence of Fire, of which the deity Agni is the ruler.
Traipura. The passive triangle at the centre of the first chakra, muladhara chakra.
Trishnâ. Desire.

U

Udhdhiriyâna Bandha. An exercise of the diaphragm.
Ujjayi. A rhythmical breathing exercise.
Unmani. One of the planes of realization beyond the mind.

V

Vaishwanara. The waking state of the human body.
Vajrâ. The name of a nâdî situated in the cerebro-spinal axis.
Vâmâchârins. Tantrik magicians.
Vârunâ. Name of a secondary nâdî.
Vâsanâ. Desire.
Vasishta. Name of a Rishi famous for his spiritual teaching ; he was the Guru of Rama.
Vâyu. The essence of the element air.

Vedântins. The school of Vedanta ; one of the most influential traditional schools of India.

Vicâra. The education of the mind.

Vijnânamaya Kosha. One of the subtile human bodies.

Vishodarâ. One of the secondary nâdîs.

Vishuddha chakra. The chakra of the throat.

Y

Yamimâ. One of the sacred rivers of India.

Yashasvani. One of the secondary nâdîs.

Yoni. Feminine, passive symbolism.

Yonimudrâ. One of the postures of Yoga.

Yuktatriveni. The meeting of the three sacred rivers of India, symbolizing the union of the three principal nâdîs.

Quality Paperbacks From Samuel Weiser

THE SECRETS OF CHINESE MEDITATION by Charles Luk.
There is no more helpful book so far as the Chinese methods are concerned than this treatise. The instructions seem to come alive and are useful.

THE HEART OF BUDDHIST MEDITATION by Nyanaponika Thera.
A handbook of mental training based on the Buddha's way of mindfulness.

THE PSYCHOLOGICAL ATTITUDE OF EARLY BUDDHIST PHILOSOPHY by Lama Anagarika Govinda.
A brilliant summary of Pali Buddhist, and a logical approach to the problems of Mahayana and Tantric philosophy which grew from the principles of nonsubstantiality and inter-relatedness of all phenomena.

FOUNDATIONS OF TIBETAN MYSTICISM by Lama Anagarika Govinda.
A masterly book on the mantra—OM MANI PADME HUM!

THE THEORY & PRACTICE OF THE MANDALA by Professor Giuseppe Tucci.
A description of the complex arrangements of the Mandalas or patterns used in Hindu and Buddhist Tantrism to express the infinite possibilities of the human subconscious.

THE COLLECTED WORKS OF RAMANA MAHARSHI edited by Arthur Osborne.
The whole book is a distillation of the doctrine and practice of Advaita or non-duality by one who had realized and renewed it in his person.

RAMANA MAHARSHI & THE PATH OF SELF-KNOWLEDGE by Arthur Osborne.
An attractive picture of one who belonged to the true line of India's spiritual teachers.

HATHA YOGA by Theos Bernard.
Copious explanations based on original sources, make this work useful to aspiring novices.

A SEARCH IN SECRET INDIA by Paul Brunton.
Those who are interested in the Eastern Science of Yoga and its practitioners will have great interest in this work.

A SEARCH IN SECRET EGYPT by Paul Brunton.
An extraordinary experience among the fakirs, snake charmers and magicians of modern Egypt.

THE WISDOM OF THE OVERSELF by Paul Brunton.
This is a complete review of the problems of those engaged in mentalist study.

THE FINDING OF THE THIRD EYE by Vera Stanley Alder.
An indication of the true path to an understanding and mastery of life.

THE INITIATION OF THE WORLD by Vera Stanley Alder.
An outline of the history of evolution according to the Ancient Wisdom, and a synthesis with the findings of modern science.

THE PROJECTION OF THE ASTRAL BODY by Sylvan Muldoon & Hereward Carrington.
A remarkable account of Sylvan Muldoon's 'out of the body' experiences.

THE PHENOMENA OF ASTRAL PROJECTION by Sylvan Muldoon & Hereward Carrington.
The collected and documented material relating to over 100 cases of astral projection.

TRANSCENDENTAL MAGIC by Eliphas Levi, translated by A. E. Waite.
Maintaining its supreme position in the field, this book covers almost the entire realm of Ritual and High Magic.